DEMENTIA SURVIVAL GUIDE FOR CAREGIVERS

UNLEASH THE POWER OF COMPASSIONATE
CAREGIVING TO CREATE HARMONY,
UNDERSTANDING, AND A STRONGER BOND WITH
YOUR LOVED ONE

OLIVER MONTCLAIR

© **Copyright 2023 - All rights reserved.**

The content contained within this book may not be reproduced, duplicated or transmitted without direct written permission from the author or the publisher.

Under no circumstances will any blame or legal responsibility be held against the publisher, or author, for any damages, reparation, or monetary loss due to the information contained within this book, either directly or indirectly.

Legal Notice:

This book is copyright protected. It is only for personal use. You cannot amend, distribute, sell, use, quote or paraphrase any part, or the content within this book, without the consent of the author or publisher.

Disclaimer Notice:

Please note the information contained within this document is for educational and entertainment purposes only. All effort has been executed to present accurate, up to date, reliable, complete information. No warranties of any kind are declared or implied. Readers acknowledge that the author is not engaged in the rendering of legal, financial, medical or professional advice. The content within this book has been derived from various sources. Please consult a licensed professional before attempting any techniques outlined in this book.

By reading this document, the reader agrees that under no circumstances is the author responsible for any losses, direct or indirect, that are incurred as a result of the use of the information contained within this document, including, but not limited to, errors, omissions, or inaccuracies.

CONTENTS

Introduction   5

1. THE MYSTERIES OF DEMENTIA   13
   A Better Understanding of Dementia   14
   How Dementia Affects Daily Life   19
   Types and Stages of Dementia   24
   The Seven Stages of Dementia   27
   Symptoms and Behavioral Changes   28

2. YOUR JOURNEY AS A CAREGIVER   35
   The Rollercoaster That Is Caregiving   37
   Introduction to the CARE+ Model   43
   Interactive Element: Self-Assessment Questionnaire   45

3. THE POWER OF COMPASSIONATE COMMUNICATION   49
   The CARE+ Model: Communication   50

4. MORE THAN JUST DAILY ACTIVITIES   69
   The CARE+ Model: Activities   70

5. RESTING YOUR HEART   97
   The CARE+ Model: Rest and Resilience   98

6. HOME, SWEET HOME   109
   The CARE+ Model: Environment   110
   Interactive Element: Home Safety Checklist   122

7. FOR YOUR PEACE OF MIND   125
   The CARE+ Model: Legal and Financial Considerations   126
   Key Tips for Dementia Caregivers   138

8. LOOKING AHEAD 139
The CARE+ Model: Care Options and End-
of-Life Care 140

Conclusion 149
References 155

INTRODUCTION

Many people know about dementia and Alzheimer's, but what's not too well-known is what caregivers go through while they help their loved ones. When President Ronald Reagan received an Alzheimer's disease diagnosis in 1994, his wife, Nancy Reagan, became his primary caregiver. She wasn't silent about the experience and brought much-needed attention to her role, which helped de-stigmatize dementia. She raised awareness about the disease and promoted research for treatment options, bringing attention to how dementia impacts the individual affected as well as their families.

Nancy Reagan's advocacy helped so many people, including myself. When a loved one received the same diagnosis as President Reagan, I knew I would step up to be their caregiver. While I love my family and would do anything for them, I soon realized that caregiving was more intense than I had anticipated. After going through that experience, I understood how crucial a guidebook could be in empowering other people who take on this same role. At times, it can feel almost impossible to care for your loved one, advocate for their medical rights, and still maintain your own life. However, after managing all of that, I wanted to share what I had learned along the way. My experience, paired with what Nancy Reagan went through and how she paved the way for others, helped me see that being a caregiver is one of the most significant roles you can take on in your life, and it should not be taken lightly.

Dementia is a group of cognitive deficits relating to the mental process involved in and affecting memory, reasoning, learning, understanding, behavior and the capacity to do daily tasks. It's related to Alzheimer's disease, vascular dementia, and Lewy body dementia. The brain's cells lose the ability to communicate with each other, causing memory loss. They may forget who you are, things from their past, and how to perform everyday tasks. This makes caregiving complex and difficult and includes providing physical, emotional, and psychological support to dementia patients. You'll need to assist patients with daily tasks they now struggle with due to cognitive deterioration. These responsibilities might range from assisting with personal cleanliness, clothing, and eating to managing medications, appointments, and finances. Caregivers play a crucial role in providing a safe and supportive environment, maintaining a structured schedule, and adapting to the evolving needs and challenges of individuals with dementia.

Caring for someone with dementia can be emotionally taxing because their personality and behavior can change over time. Caregivers may experience feelings of irritation, guilt, grief, and even burnout due to the ongoing demands of the role. Additionally, the person with dementia may experience agitation, disorientation, and anxiety, making the caregiving task even more complicated. It's not uncommon for caregivers to find themselves at odds with the person they care for, even though they wish they could be more patient and understanding. It can be challenging to manage someone at this level when you have such a personal connection with them.

Patience, empathy, and understanding are required for effective dementia caregiving. Caregivers must learn to communicate in ways that take into account the person's cognitive capacities as well as changes in language skills. Creating a consistent and supportive environment can aid in reducing anxiety and improving general well-being. However, you need to balance that with your needs and emotions, which can be difficult when you're caring for a friend or family member. At times, they may be unable to remember your name or relationship, and while it's simply a result of the dementia, it can really hurt your feelings. It can be a struggle to remain neutral and continue caring for them, but it's essential to do so for their well-being and your own.

There has been a rising realization in recent years of the necessity of helping dementia carers. Education, respite care, counseling, and access to community resources are all forms of assistance. Caregivers are encouraged to seek aid and maintain their own physical and mental health in order to continue providing the best possible care to their dementia-affected patients. I hope to use my research and experience to help those who are taking on this challenging role.

I never envisaged becoming a full-time caretaker for my loved one, who was diagnosed with Alzheimer's disease. Growing up, this person was our family's rock, full of wisdom and stories. However, their memory and personality began to fade as the disease worsened. The indicators were modest initially, such as misplaced keys or forgotten appointments, but it eventually became evident that something was wrong. My family and I were thrown into dementia caregiving, which required us to adapt, learn, and support one another in ways we never expected.

During my time as a caregiver, I experienced the emotional ups and downs of the job. I often had to deal with my loved one asking the same question repeatedly within a short period. I learned to be patient and respond to their queries with a smile, even if I had just answered the same question moments ago. It was difficult to watch their fading health, but I was there to provide the care and support they needed.

Witnessing their fading memory was one of the most challenging things. They struggled to recognize me at times, and each time they inquired who I was, it felt like a dagger to the heart. But then there were those rare occasions when my loved one's eyes would light up, and they would call me by name, sharing a recollection from our past. Those were like beams of sunshine breaking through the clouds, reminding me of the robust and lively person they used to be.

The difficulties go beyond memory loss. My loved one's actions became more erratic and unpredictable, causing them to shift from a state of laughter to agitation or anxiety in seconds. It was heartbreaking to see them struggle with simple tasks like buttoning a shirt or tying shoelaces, which had once been effortless. The frustration with the inability to care for themselves made them irritable, causing them to lash out at me. It was difficult not to take their outbursts personally, but I knew it was the disease, not my family member, causing this behavior.

My family, friends, and support groups were my lifelines during these challenging times. Speaking with people going through similar circumstances made me feel less alone and better prepared to face the obstacles. Additionally, respite care allowed me to regroup and take care of myself, which I realized was critical to me offering the best care.

During the process, I learned to value the small triumphs achieved along the way, such as the coy smiles, bonding, and the enjoyable moments we still shared. This experience taught me the importance of patience and humility and the power of unconditional love. Despite the numerous obstacles, I wouldn't exchange the time I spent looking after my loved one for anything.

Of course, their condition deteriorated further over time. We had to make the difficult decision to place them in a specialized care facility at some point. Knowing they would receive the round-the-clock care required while understanding the progression's finality was a bittersweet moment.

Caring for a family member with dementia was a life-altering experience that completely changed my perspective on family, compassion, and the significance of each moment. It was a journey that will always remain etched in my memory, a testament to the bravery and resilience caregivers exhibit when confronted with life's toughest challenges. Initially, I assumed that caregiving would be a natural process, but it turned out to be much more complicated than I had expected. Although I cherished the time I spent taking care of my loved one, I also realized that I acquired a lot of knowledge about them, dementia, and myself, and I can share those lessons to make this journey easier for others who are going through the same situation.

I follow the CARE+ model, which is a holistic approach to compassionate caregiving. This model focuses on compassionate **communication, activities** for daily care, **rest and resilience** for the caregiver, and a supportive **environment, plus** other considerations, such as legal and financial issues. The structured framework gives you everything you need to manage this challenging time, offering guidance and support as you care for your loved one, their home and legacy. The CARE+ model aims to make caregiving a more compassionate experience, allowing you to support your loved one without losing yourself in the process and promoting meaningful interactions while they are still possible. Each chapter of this book covers core concepts, including background information on dementia and becoming a caregiver, as well as adjusting to life after supporting your loved one.

1

THE MYSTERIES OF DEMENTIA

Kindness can transform someone's dark moment with a blaze of light. You'll never know how much your caring matters. Make a difference for another day.

— AMY LEIGH MERCREE

The human brain, with its sophisticated and intricate web of neuronal connections, serves as the center of our ideas, memories, and identities. However, despite the wonders of cognition, dementia casts a profound shadow over the mind's brilliance. This disease presents a multitude of puzzles that continue to perplex scientists, physicians, and families alike. As the world's population ages and the frequency of dementia increases, its perplexing characteristics receive growing attention.

The researchers are currently delving deeper into the origins, processes, and potential treatments of dementia. The condition poses a significant challenge that extends far beyond medicine. Given the intricate nature of the brain, it forces us to contemplate the very essence of what it means to be human. Rather than attempting to solve the mysteries of dementia, this book will explore the layers of the brain, in an attempt to comprehend the inexplicable. It is essential to understand the mysteries of dementia before assuming the role of a caregiver. This will enable you to comprehend what their experiencing and adjust your care methods accordingly.

A BETTER UNDERSTANDING OF DEMENTIA

Dementia is often considered a distinct disease, but it is a syndrome that encompasses a range of symptoms affecting memory, thought processes, communication, and behavior. Understanding the nature of this syndrome and how it presents in individuals can provide valuable insight into what your loved one is experiencing and how you can best support them.

What Is Dementia?

Dementia is a condition where cognitive function declines, making it challenging for patients to carry out daily activities. This decline is often caused by damage to or death of brain cells, which impairs normal brain function. As a result, patients may struggle to participate in activities they once found easy and may require assistance with daily tasks.

Dementia is a condition that affects the brain and causes a decline in cognitive function. The most common cause of dementia is Alzheimer's disease, which is also the most prevalent type. However, dementia can also be caused by other factors, such as reduced blood flow to the brain, known as vascular dementia. Another type of dementia, Lewy body dementia, is caused by abnormal protein deposits in the brain. Frontotemporal dementia affects the frontal and temporal lobes of the brain. Apart from these, there are other causes of dementia, which will be discussed in detail later in this chapter.

Dementia is a condition that gradually worsens over time. Unfortunately, there is currently no cure for it. However, early detection and effective management strategies can enhance the quality of life for patients. Various treatments may help manage the symptoms and facilitate lifestyle adjustments.

How Prevalent Is It?

Dementia is a significant global health concern that affects the elderly population. Its prevalence varies worldwide depending on demographics, access to healthcare, education, and awareness. According to the World Health

Organization (2023), more than 55 million people have dementia, and approximately 10 million new cases are diagnosed yearly. As the baby boomer population ages, the cases are expected to increase. Research shows that people with higher education levels are less likely to develop dementia. In a 2019 study, only 5% of older adults with a college degree had dementia, while 18% of individuals with less than 12 years of education had the condition (Population Reference Bureau, 2023).

Dementia is a condition that affects older people, with the highest percentage of cases found in adults aged 90 or older. It is more common in women than men, and people of color are more likely to develop it than white adults (Population Reference Bureau, 2023). However, dementia is often underdiagnosed, particularly in its early stages. Many people attribute forgetfulness or a busy mind to aging, and this casual approach to the early signs means that some individuals do not seek medical attention until the condition has progressed. This lowers their chances of receiving effective interventions and skews the statistics regarding diagnosis. Regardless of when people receive a dementia diagnosis, it is projected that the number of dementia cases will increase significantly, reaching an estimated 82 million by 2030 and more than 152 million by 2050 (World Health Organization, 2023).

It may be surprising to learn that despite the staggering statistics, people with dementia are four times more likely to live in their own homes than residential care, according to the Population Reference Bureau in 2023. As a result, many caregivers need to understand this condition and learn how to help them live a comfortable life as they age.

Caring for someone with dementia can be demanding. Due to the high cost of nursing homes and residential care, most people with dementia rely on their family members as unpaid caregivers. Even if your loved one moves into an assisted living facility, they may still have unpaid caregivers checking in on them to ensure they are doing well in the new environment. Statistics highlight the challenges of caring for someone with dementia.

A Brief History of Dementia Research

Dementia research has been developing over the years, as more people have been experiencing this condition and medical professionals have been searching for potential treatments. The condition was first recorded in the early 19th century, describing the mental decline older people experience as they age (Assal, 2019). However, there wasn't any research or possible cause.

In the early 20th century, German psychologist Alois Alzheimer began researching dementia. Specifically, his work on a patient named Auguste Deter helped him identify brain tangles and plaques that are now known to signify Alzheimer's disease (Neundörfer, 2003).

By the mid-20th century, researchers started to notice the differences between Alzheimer's disease and other types of dementia, like vascular and frontotemporal (Assal, 2019).

The late 20th century saw great advancements in dementia research. First, there were advancements in imaging that helped researchers notice structural brain changes in people with dementia (Patel et al., 2020). Doctors were able to identify biomarkers associated with various forms of dementia, like beta-amyloid and tau proteins representing Alzheimer's disease (Bloom, 2014). This information also paved the way for genetic insights, like APOE4, associated with an increased risk of Alzheimer's disease (Bryant, 2021).

By the beginning of the 21st century, researchers began developing medications that targeted dementia symptoms, like cholinesterase inhibitors that help manage cognitive decline, though nothing could provide a cure (Singh & Sadiq, 2023). However, along with medication research, medical professionals found that some lifestyle factors could reduce the risk of dementia, such as a healthy diet, exercise, social interaction, and cognitive stimulation.

Currently, many ongoing clinical trials test new drugs and interventions for dementia. Researchers noticed commonalities between dementia, Parkinson's disease, and amyotrophic lateral sclerosis (ALS) and broadened their studies to improve their ability to detect biomarkers in individuals. This field expansion increases the potential to develop targeted therapies for specific dementia subtypes, which offers hope for more effective treatments in the future.

HOW DEMENTIA AFFECTS DAILY LIFE

Dementia is a progressive condition that starts slowly and creeps up on the patient. It often begins with small things, like forgetting where they left their keys or blanking on someone's name, even when that person is right in front of them. As the condition worsens, people may lose their short-term memory. This can lead to forgetting necessary appointments, names, and conversations and needing help remembering why they went to a particular location.

As the condition progresses, patients may also have difficulty communicating. Finding the right words can be a challenge, whether recalling a specific term from their past or simply naming a common kitchen appliance they use daily. Many dementia patients feel embarrassed by their inability to express themselves, which may cause them to withdraw socially. They may feel it's better to be isolated than to have others see them struggle for words.

Patients with dementia face difficulty in finding the right words, which is a sign of their inability to make decisions. They can struggle to solve problems that they previously could solve with ease. They may have trouble planning their daily activities and fail to think critically while scheduling events. They can make mistakes when managing their finances or preparing meals independently.

All of these issues contribute to the disorientation that people with dementia experience. They feel disconnected from themselves and are unable to remember where they are or why they are there. They lose track of time and may not know what day it is. Even if they are in their familiar neighborhood, they may not remember the directions to leave the house and walk down the street to the corner store.

Many individuals who suffer from dementia experience behavioral changes as the condition progresses due to the mental disruptions it causes. They might feel frustrated that they cannot remember things or complete tasks that were once easy for them. After being able to live independently, they may lash out at caregivers because they dislike being dependent on someone else. They may also experience difficulty falling and staying asleep, leading to exhaustion and confusion.

These symptoms together can lead to dementia patients withdrawing from society. They may be embarrassed about their inability to perform certain tasks or remember things and may not want their friends to see them in this state. They may also face challenges with hygiene, bathing, and using the bathroom, which can make them prefer staying home instead of going out.

Dementia can lead to confusion and forgetfulness, which increase the safety risks associated with simple tasks. For instance, cooking meals can be challenging for dementia patients because they might forget to check the oven when food is baking and burn it. They may also overlook turning off the burner, causing a fire. People with dementia patients may accidentally lock themselves out of their homes and wander off in search of help, forgetting where they are and who they are in the process.

It is important to note that not all dementia patients experience the same symptoms or at the same severity levels. Some people may experience a rapid decline, while others may maintain their memories and actions for a longer period of time.

Why Caregivers Need to Understand Dementia

Caregivers must understand dementia in order to provide the best possible support. This knowledge is essential to offer the right care and manage the challenges that arise as their condition worsens. Knowing as much as possible about dementia will also help you anticipate what may happen and take the necessary steps to ensure that you and your loved one can handle all the twists and turns that come with this diagnosis.

One of the most important things to note about dementia is how it causes communication difficulties. They may not be able to express themselves accurately. For instance, they might forget your name or refer to a coffee pot as a "drink-making thing." If you know this will happen, you can pay close attention to what they are saying, including reading their body language, to help them feel understood.

As their behavior may change, you should brace yourself for mood swings, agitation, aggression, and withdrawal. Since you're caring for a loved one, it can be hard not to take these behaviors personally. However, you must remember that their actions result from dementia, not how they truly feel. You'll be better able to regulate your emotions when you keep this in mind, instead of feeling too emotionally invested in in their current behaviors. You should respond empathetically, putting your loved one first, instead of being wrapped up in your feelings.

When you put your loved one first, you'll prioritize a safe environment for them. Eliminate risks to their health and safety, such as identifying fall hazards and safeguarding locks, cabinets, and dangerous appliances. If they're on medication, know the schedules and possible side effects, and ensure they take their medicines as directed. You can use a daily pill tray to dispense their medications if they can take them independently, and keep track of how many pills are left so you can tell if they took their daily dose or too many. You will also want to communicate with their medical team so everyone is on the same page regarding the symptoms, severity, and possible treatment plans and interventions. You'll want to be an advocate, helping them maintain their independence for as long as possible while keeping them safe and comfortable, with the respect they deserve.

While a lot of caregiving will involve medication and symptom management, you can also enjoy time with them. Meaningful activities may help them remember who they are and what they love. You can also help boost their brain power by doing puzzles and playing games together. Some dementia patients enjoy looking at photo albums, even if they don't remember everyone in the pictures. You may want to read aloud or go on walks to get fresh air, ensuring you help them stay steady on their feet and prevent them from getting lost.

As a caregiver, you'll need to understand coping strategies for yourself. It's a lot to take on, especially as it's mentally, emotionally, and physically demanding unpaid labor. However, you'll also want to help them cope. You can be patient and understanding with them so they don't feel as anxious or confused when you're with them. You can help them mitigate these symptoms to improve their quality of life. You might want to keep them independent by assisting only slightly, like laying out clothes and helping them button shirts or precooking ingredients and letting them mix them to finish the meal.

Understanding dementia helps you anticipate your own emotional needs while also helping your loved one live their best life regardless of their cognitive state. Being aware of all aspects of the condition will help you prioritize their health, while also managing your self-care and support so you're strong enough to handle the caregiving role.

TYPES AND STAGES OF DEMENTIA

Dementia is the name for a group of progressive cognitive disorders that impact memory, thoughts, behavior, and physical abilities. There are many types of dementia, and each has unique characteristics, symptoms, and causes. There are also stages of dementia that reference the progression of the symptoms.

Alzheimer's Disease

Alzheimer's disease is the most common form of dementia, characterized by the accumulation of abnormal brain proteins such as beta-amyloid plaques and tau tangles. Symptoms of Alzheimer's disease may include:

- confusion
- difficulty communicating
- inability to care for self
- memory loss
- restlessness and agitation
- shortened attention span
- withdrawal from social activities (National Institute on Aging, 2022)

Vascular Dementia

Vascular dementia is caused by reduced oxygen and blood flow to the brain, which happens due to strokes or small vessel disease that creates vascular issues. These issues can be visible on MRI scans. However, it's important to note that not everyone who has a stroke is at risk for vascular dementia. Symptoms of this type of dementia may include:

- changes in personality and behavior
- difficulty completing common tasks
- forgetfulness
- hallucinations and delusions
- inability to follow instructions
- loss of interest in hobbies and family
- struggling to find the correct word (National Institute on Aging, 2021a)

Lewy Body Dementia

Lewy body dementia is characterized by the presence of abnormal protein deposits in the brain, known as Lewy bodies. The symptoms, which include those similar to Alzheimer's and Parkinson's, can make it challenging to diagnose initially. Symptoms include:

- confusion about times and places
- difficulty remembering words and numbers

- inability to concentrate or stay alert
- physical issues like stiffness, slow movement, and repeated falls
- poor judgment
- tremors in extremities that can impact handwriting and simple tasks
- visual hallucinations (National Institute on Aging, 2021c)

Frontotemporal Dementia

Frontotemporal dementia is a condition that affects the frontal and temporal lobes of the brain. These areas play an important role in shaping our personality, language, and behavior. There are two distinct types of frontotemporal dementia, depending on the changes that occur in the brain. One type is called behavioral variant FTD (bvFTD). It can cause problems with planning and sequencing. For example, patients may repeat the same word or do the same action over and over without being able to stop.

The other type is known as primary progressive aphasia (PPA), which greatly impacts the ability to communicate. People with PPA have trouble reading, writing, speaking, and understanding what others say to them. They may slur their speech or become mute. In the early stages of PPA, individuals may lose some of their language, drop words from sentences, or forget specific words in a conversation (National Institute on Aging, 2017a).

Mixed Dementia

When an individual has more than one type of dementia, it is referred to as mixed dementia. The most common types of dementia are Alzheimer's disease and vascular dementia, but there can be various combinations of these conditions. It can be challenging to diagnose the specific type of dementia as many of them have similar symptoms. Hence, it may require extensive testing and medical intervention to determine the appropriate treatment.

THE SEVEN STAGES OF DEMENTIA

Medical professionals use stages to represent the severity and progressive nature of dementia. Although the stages may present differently in each individual, they generally follow a pattern.

Stage 1 indicates no cognitive decline. Your loved one appears to have the same cognitive function as always.

Stage 2 is a very mild cognitive decline and is characterized by minor memory lapses such as forgetting a name or word, which may be a normal part of aging.

Stage 3 is a mild cognitive decline characterized by noticeable difficulties in concentration and memory. This may be the first time that family members or the loved one become aware of changes in their abilities.

Stage 4 is a moderate cognitive decline. They may struggle with complex tasks and forget things that just happened. They're unable to drive or travel independently and may struggle with their finances.

Stage 5 is a moderately severe cognitive decline. More help with daily tasks will be required. They may also experience broader gaps in their memory and forget their personal past.

Stage 6 is a severe cognitive decline. This can include difficulty remembering names, displaying personality changes, and requiring constant supervision.

Stage 7 is a severe cognitive decline, the final stage of dementia. They may have difficulty communicating, walking, sitting, and holding up their head. It's important to provide extensive support to keep them comfortable at home, as per Reed-Guy (2013).

SYMPTOMS AND BEHAVIORAL CHANGES

Dementia causes various cognitive, emotional, and behavioral changes in individuals. The symptoms and intensity may differ depending on the specific diagnosis and situation of the person affected (National Institute on Aging, 2021b). Knowing the general signs of dementia is essential to providing the necessary support. This way, you can ensure that they receive the appropriate care they need to manage their condition.

Memory Loss

Dementia is a condition that primarily affects memory. One of the major signs of dementia is memory loss, where an individual may find it difficult to recall recent events or conversations. This can lead to repetitive questioning, where they ask the same question repeatedly, even if they have been answered before. Additionally, people with dementia may forget their daily routine tasks like appointments or the way to their favorite place in the neighborhood.

Cognitive Decline

With any type of dementia, you will notice a decline in cognitive abilities. Initially, the decline may not be very noticeable, but it will progress significantly as time passes. Your loved one will have difficulty with reasoning and problem-solving skills and may struggle to keep things organized or plan tasks that were previously effortless for them. As their caregiver, you will want to provide guidance, but they may struggle to understand your instructions and follow them accurately.

Communication Difficulties

As individuals with memory loss progress, they may also experience a decline in their language abilities. They may find it difficult to recall the names of everyday objects and struggle to articulate their own thoughts due to limited vocabulary. Eventually, they may face challenges in understanding your communication and body language, which can lead to misunderstandings and conflicts.

Disorientation

It's important to understand that disorientation can affect both physical and mental states. Your loved one may become confused about the weather patterns of different seasons and may call you by the name of their parent or may not recognize you at all. They may find it difficult to remember correct times and dates. They may also get lost in familiar places, and may struggle to recall locations that were significant to them earlier in their life.

Behavioral and Mood Changes

Dealing with dementia can be challenging as it can cause changes in behavior and mood that vary from person to person. Some individuals may not experience significant changes since they were already expressive in their emotions. On the other hand, even those who were reserved may exhibit mood swings and emotional instability that may come as a surprise. Memory issues can make them feel irritable and cause them to withdraw from social interactions.

Trouble With Routine Tasks

Dementia can cause individuals to forget how to perform basic tasks and lose control of their fingers and extremities, which can affect their ability to dress, bathe, and groom themselves. Additionally, individuals with dementia may pose a safety risk if they try to cook or use appliances.

Inability to Recognize Faces

Watching memory loss can be challenging. One of the most difficult symptoms is the trouble they may have in recognizing faces. Even if you see them every day, they may forget your name and the relationship you share with them. They may mistake family members for strangers. Remember that this is not personal, and it is important to be patient and understanding.

Changes in Sleep Patterns

As cognitive decline worsens, sleep patterns may change with insomnia or they may nap during at random times the during the day.

Wandering and Restlessness

It is possible that the change in sleep patterns is connected to the increase in wandering and restlessness. They may walk around the house aimlessly or pace, and attempt to leave the house. It is important to prioritize their safety in these instances. Clear all paths and ensure there are no carpets or rugs that may cause them to trip. Additionally, it is crucial to lock all doors and windows securely and consider installing a security system that alerts you whenever a door is opened.

Hallucinations and Delusions

As the brain structure changes, they may start experiencing hallucinations wherein they see, hear, or sense things that don't actually exist. These hallucinations may seem very real to them, but you won't be able to perceive anything unusual. They may also develop delusions or false beliefs about things, such as believing that you're stealing money from them when in reality, they simply misplaced a check and can't recall where they kept it.

Appetite Changes

As a person with dementia progresses, they may fall into a pattern of overeating or forgetting to eat, leading to weight gain or loss. As a caregiver, it's important to monitor their eating habits and help them maintain a healthy diet. You can prepare pre-portioned, nutritious meals for them and ensure they eat at scheduled mealtimes to keep them physically healthy. A balanced diet can be instrumental in keeping their bowel movements regular, which is important for their overall well-being.

Aggression and Agitation

As a result of cognitive changes, your loved one may become more aggressive and agitated. They may feel uncomfortable or overwhelmed easily since nothing feels familiar to them anymore. Dementia can also cause incontinence, as your loved one struggles to control their bladder and bowel. This can lead to feelings of embarrassment or anger, which may result in outbursts of frustration. Furthermore, their changed behavior may cause them to lose their sense of social etiquette and react impulsively, leading to a lack of awareness of social norms.

2

YOUR JOURNEY AS A CAREGIVER

Caregiving often calls us to lean into love we didn't know possible.

— TIA WALKER

Caregivers of loved ones with dementia face more challenges than you'd initially imagine. Caring for others is always demanding, taxing you emotionally, physically, and mentally. However, it's painful to see when you're caring for someone you love who is experiencing such a degenerative condition. Your family member goes through changes in their memory, behavior, and cognitive abilities. As the disease progresses, you do more and more to keep them comfortable, to the extent that you often overlook your own needs.

As dementia progresses, it can affect the ability to communicate, making it harder for you to understand their wants and needs. This can lead to conflicts and frustrations for both of you. The inability to communicate can leave you both feeling helpless and struggling to understand each other.

It is important to note that as a caregiver, you may experience changes in your loved one's behavior. They may seem like a different person and exhibit unusual behaviors such as spacing out during conversations and wandering off. They may also become easily frustrated and agitated, leading to aggressive actions. It can be challenging to manage these behaviors because your loved one is an adult used to living independently without close oversight.

Caregiving can be a very difficult and emotional experience. Even if you have nurses to assist you, witnessing emotional and physical decline can be overwhelming. The person you once knew so well may no longer be the same, and it can be heartbreaking. Dementia patients may also experience grief for the loss of their previous quality of life during rare moments of clarity. They are gradually losing their memories and cognitive abilities which greatly contribute to their uniqueness and enjoyment of life.

Taking on the role of a caregiver can be emotionally challenging. However, it's important to balance these common emotions with the benefits of caregiving. If you feel overwhelmed, don't worry. The CARE+ model is available to guide you every step of the way and offer the support you need. By showing love when your family member needs it most, you'll feel empowered and fulfilled.

THE ROLLERCOASTER THAT IS CAREGIVING

Caring for loved ones with conditions like dementia can be an emotionally challenging and difficult process. It can be a rollercoaster ride with a range of experiences and problems that may come as a surprise when you take on the role. As a caregiver, you have to provide physical, emotional, and sometimes even financial support while navigating the unexpected twists and turns that come with the job. Understanding the emotional landscape of caregiving, identifying common emotions experienced by caregivers, and highlighting some unexpected benefits that can result from it will help you prepare for the challenges you may encounter when you take on this responsibility.

Common Emotions in Caregiving

As a caregiver, you are an unsung hero providing unwavering support. Love is at the foundation of your work. It's the reason you do what you do, often sacrificing your own needs to put your loved one first. You demonstrate love by making meals for your family member to ensure they eat and keep up their strength. You touch them with love when you bathe them to help them feel clean and comfortable despite the complications of dementia.

As a caregiver, love is at the center of your commitment. You may experience feelings of being overwhelmed and distressed, but you know that the family bond is so strong that you couldn't consider any other option regarding their care. However, this can lead to frustration. It can be frustrating when your they can't remember their own name and you are left to manage all their appointments, medications, and more. It can often feel like you're trapped in a never-ending cycle of managing their life with no break.

Providing nonstop care can be overwhelming and exhausting. You may feel mentally and physically drained most of the time, as you need to provide care at any given moment, and as the condition worsens, you may need to provide care around the clock. Due to stress or staying awake to assist with insomnia, you may not get enough sleep.

Every task you complete holds a glimmer of hope. The hope that you are making life a little better for your loved one. The hope that they will remember your name or share a memory from their childhood. This hope may be intertwined with sorrow and grief, but its presence is a testament to the fact that you are doing things for the right reasons.

Providing care is a turbulent emotional experience that can leave you feeling a range of mood swings, despite the desire to stay rational.

Being a caregiver is not an easy task. It can be overwhelming and you might experience waves of guilt and self-doubt. You might feel uncertain about the decisions you're making and wonder if it's what's best for your loved one. Even if you're already doing everything you can, you may still feel guilty for not doing enough. These emotions can be triggered by tough decisions about medical care, finances, or living arrangements.

In addition to guilt and doubt, you may also experience frustration and helplessness. It can be frustrating to see the decline and not be able to do anything about it. You might feel helpless when you can't communicate and decode their message, making you even more frustrated. It's important to remember that these are normal emotions and that you need to be patient and adapt to help them in their new state.

As you embark on your caregiving journey, you will inevitably experience feelings of sadness and grief. It can be emotionally draining to witness the gradual deterioration of mind and body, and while you may be spending more time with them to help maintain their independence, it can take a toll on you. Additionally, the patient themselves may experience a sense of loss and grief over who they once were, and in moments of clarity, they may realize what is happening to their brain and body, which can be very difficult to cope with. It is essential to recognize that caring for someone during this time is not easy, and it is okay to feel overwhelmed by these emotions. Therefore, it is crucial to be kind to yourself and allow yourself the time and space to navigate through these emotions.

Being a caregiver dealing with a debilitating illness like dementia is a massive task that can cause stress and anxiety. With so much uncertainty surrounding their condition, it's normal to feel worried and anxious about their safety and medical needs. Despite having a great medical team on your side, you may still feel uneasy about what the future holds, including how long they can continue living at home and what kind of treatments will help alleviate some of their symptoms.

As a caregiver, your primary focus is on the safety and well-being of your loved one. This means that other aspects of your life, such as self-care and socializing, may be put on hold. You may feel isolated and lonely because it can be challenging to juggle other relationships while being a caregiver. It's also possible that you don't feel like you have a support network because everyone depends on you.

All these emotions can build up and cause you to feel angry and resentful. It's not uncommon to feel frustrated and resentful about the situation, the illness itself, and even the one you're caring for. However, feeling these emotions doesn't mean you hate your family member or wish you weren't caring for them. It's important to understand that it's normal to feel this way due to the immense pressure you're under. So, don't let these feelings result in more guilt on your behalf.

Benefits of Caregiving

As you read through the emotions commonly experienced by caregivers, you may question whether taking on this responsibility is the right choice for you. Remember that taking on this role can bring incredible benefits, even though you may experience a wide range of emotions.

Caring for a loved one can be emotionally challenging, but it can also bring you closer to them and create lasting memories. In moments of clarity, they will appreciate your efforts, so hold on to that knowledge.

Taking care of a family member can bring about personal growth. Even medical professionals are surprised by how much they learn about themselves while providing care. This experience can help you develop traits such as patience, problem-solving skills, adaptability, and resilience.

Taking care of someone with dementia can change your perspective on life. It can reveal how sheltered or inexperienced you may have been before the experience. You can learn harsh truths about human behavior and the fragility of life on a different level. It can make you reevaluate your priorities and develop a new appreciation for the present moments.

Despite the difficulties that come with caregiving, the biggest benefit is the sense of fulfillment it brings. Although some days may be incredibly trying and exhausting, the feeling of being able to be a caregiver can be gratifying. It's a chance to give back and show gratitude for all the love they have given you over the years. Knowing you can provide love and care to someone who means so much to you can keep you going daily.

You may come across a supportive community and reliable support pillars to assist you in your particular circumstance. Some families come together to take on the caregiving role in shifts so that they can share the burden and spend quality time with their family member. You may have access to dementia support groups and resources in your locality. These resources allow you to validate your experience, share advice, and listen to your thoughts and feelings. Having the support of those who have gone through similar experiences can help you grasp the magnitude of what you are doing. If you don't have such support in person, that's what I aim to offer through this book.

Reading this book will not only increase your knowledge of dementia and caregiving, but it will also make you an advocate for your loved one. You'll gain a deeper understanding of the importance of standing up for dementia patients and raising awareness of this condition. You can also support research efforts to find a cure for this disease.

Caregivers display unwavering love and commitment despite the emotional turmoil involved in the task. Their dedication is a testament to the human spirit and its resilience. They face stress and adversity daily, yet they charge forth as caregivers to provide everything they can for their loved ones. That's why the CARE+ model is so important.

INTRODUCTION TO THE CARE+ MODEL

The CARE+ model is an all-encompassing approach to caregiving that prioritizes the needs of both the caregiver and the patient. This unique method provides a supportive environment for everyone affected by dementia diagnosis, with a structured framework to help you and your family navigate the complex challenges of dementia care. While you may have come across some information from dementia resources, the CARE+ model offers a comprehensive approach that focuses on both the patient and the caregiver. Dementia patients face medical issues, while caregivers provide love, support, and medical attention. Considering the bigger picture, it's evident that everyone involved needs support for compassionate caregiving. The CARE+ model is designed to meet these needs, making it easier for caregivers to support their loved ones while also caring for themselves.

This book will teach you about the core features of the CARE+ model, which include communication, activities, rest and resilience, environment, and other considerations. The goal is to enhance the quality of life for both caregivers and their loved ones, while alleviating the stress and anxiety that come with this time.

With the CARE+ model, you'll have actionable steps to follow to improve your communication skills, making your time together more meaningful. You'll also learn how to adapt their daily activities and environment to keep them safe, engaged with the world around them, and boost their confidence while slowing down cognitive decline.

As a caregiver, it's important to take care of yourself so that you can better care for others. This involves learning how to become more resilient and manage stress effectively. By doing so, you can achieve a healthy balance between your personal life and caregiving responsibilities. When you prioritize your physical and emotional well-being, you'll be better equipped to make a positive impact on your loved one's life.

Each chapter of the CARE+ model focuses on a key aspect of caregiving, helping you understand how it can benefit both you and your loved one and providing guidance on how to apply it in your daily life.

INTERACTIVE ELEMENT: SELF-ASSESSMENT QUESTIONNAIRE

Before delving into the CARE+ model, it's important to take a moment to evaluate your own condition. It's easy to get consumed by caregiving responsibilities, but neglecting your own well-being is not advisable. Taking some time to be honest with yourself and understand how you're feeling can help you identify where to focus your attention as you learn how the CARE+ model can assist you.

In the past week, I've:

Struggled to focus on my work ___ Yes ___ No

Felt guilty leaving my loved one alone ___ Yes ___ No

Struggled to make decisions ___ Yes ___ No

Felt exhausted and/or overwhelmed ___ Yes ___ No

Felt useful and appreciated ___ Yes ___ No

Felt lonely and out of touch with friends ___ Yes ___ No

I am feeling upset because the person I love has changed ___ Yes ___ No

Been upset that I have no personal time ___ Yes ___ No

Had sleep interrupted because of my caregiving tasks ___ Yes ___ No

Felt supported by other relatives ___ Yes ___ No

Worried that my loved one's home isn't safe anymore ___ Yes ___ No

Slacked on work responsibilities due to caregiving ___ Yes ___ No

Cried ___ Yes ___ No

Felt physical pain ___ Yes ___ No

Felt sick ___ Yes ___ No

Score your assessment.

To determine your level of distress, count the number of times you answered "Yes" to the questions. If you answered "Yes" to most of the questions, it is likely that you are experiencing a high level of distress. On the other hand, if you answered "No" to half or more of the questions, you might be heading towards burnout and should be cautious. Even if you answered "No" to most questions, following the CARE+ model will help you avoid getting any higher on this self-assessment.

If you are feeling highly stressed, don't worry, this book has the CARE+ model tips and resources to help you. However, talking to other family members and sharing the caregiving load is essential. You can also seek the help of social workers or medical professionals to provide relief for you. In addition, make sure to visit your doctor for an assessment to ensure that you are getting all the vitamins and nutrients you need. Remember, taking care of yourself is crucial before you can care for someone else. So, prioritize your health before we start working on improving communication.

3

THE POWER OF COMPASSIONATE COMMUNICATION

Too often we underestimate the power of a touch, a smile, a kind word, a listening ear, an honest compliment, or the smallest act of caring, all of which have the potential to turn a life around.

— LEO BUSCAGLIA

Effective communication is vital in any relationship. When you take the time to actively listen to others and engage with them, you create an open line of communication that encourages trust and strengthens your connection. When caring for someone with dementia, communication becomes even more critical. You must consider their needs and wants while balancing them with medical advice. Additionally, you must communicate with them as a family member. As their condition progresses, communicating verbally in the way you're used to becomes more challenging. This makes juggling all these communication options even more complicated than you might expect. The CARE+ model promotes compassionate communication, transforming conflicts into opportunities for connection and helping you build a deeper understanding with your loved one.

THE CARE+ MODEL: COMMUNICATION

Effective communication is crucial for individuals with dementia for multiple reasons. It enables the expression of their needs, emotions, and thoughts, which can help caregivers provide appropriate support. Good communication can also alleviate irritation and anxiety caused by confusion or unmet needs. Additionally, continuous communication helps maintain a person's sense of identity and connection to others, contributing to their overall well-being. By feeling more like their authentic selves, individuals with dementia can feel better, and their symptoms may even improve.

Communication Breakdown

As dementia progresses, communication can become increasingly challenging. Language skills may decline, making it hard to express oneself coherently, comprehend complex topics, or find the right words. Memory loss can lead to repeated questions or difficulty recalling recent events, causing conversations to become disjointed. The ability to follow discussions may also deteriorate, causing individuals to lose track of what is being said.

Dementia can cause a range of communication difficulties. People may struggle to understand abstract concepts, such as metaphors or hypothetical situations. They may also misinterpret social cues, leading to misunderstandings during social interactions. Emotional expressions may change, resulting in inappropriate laughter or tears that are unrelated to the situation at hand.

Communicating effectively can be extremely challenging, particularly in unfamiliar or noisy environments. Crowded social gatherings or public locations can be overwhelming due to sensory overload, leading to difficulty in engaging in conversations. Additionally, communication can be hindered by the effects of "sundowning," which can cause fatigue and confusion in the late afternoon or evening hours.

Dementia can impact cognitive functions that are essential for effective dialogue, such as memory, attention, logic, and problem-solving abilities. This can lead to individuals becoming more passive in conversations, finding it difficult to initiate topics, or relying on familiar phrases.

As dementia progresses, communication tends to deteriorate further. People with dementia may become more introverted and struggle to interpret language, which can result in increasing isolation and dissatisfaction.

Nonverbal communication, such as facial expressions and gestures, may also become less expressive and cohesive over time.

Several factors can influence a person's ability to communicate effectively. Their overall physical and mental health, the situation they are in, the familiarity with their surroundings, and the presence of caretakers and loved ones who understand their communication style can all play a role. By adapting communication tactics to the individual's abilities, using visual aids, and practicing patience and active listening, it is possible to improve communication.

Compassionate Communication for Caregivers

Communication will vary depending on the stage of dementia. During the early stage of dementia, they might experience mild memory lapses and difficulty finding words. You can encourage conversation by being patient. Allow time for them to think of what they're saying without trying to finish their thoughts. Pay close attention to what they're saying. Show interest and respond with empathy. Allow them to express themselves and make decisions. Respect their opinions and preferences. When you talk to them, speak slowly and use simple, straightforward language. Use visual cues like pictures, diagrams, or written instructions to enhance understanding.

Communication with a loved one with dementia requires a different approach depending on the stage of their condition. In the early stage, they may experience mild memory lapses and difficulty finding words. To encourage conversation, it's important to be patient and give them time to express themselves without interruption. Pay close attention to what they're saying, show interest, and respond with empathy. Respect their opinions and preferences, and use visual cues like pictures, diagrams, or written instructions to enhance their understanding. Speak slowly and use simple, straightforward language.

As dementia progresses, communicating verbally becomes increasingly difficult. It's important to focus on nonverbal cues and understand how to use facial expressions, eye contact, and touch to compassionately communicate. Sitting with them, staying in their line of vision, and maintaining a calm presence can provide a sense of comfort. Avoid sudden movements or approaching from outside their field of vision to prevent distress. Engage their senses with familiar objects, textures, scents, and music that can evoke memories. It's crucial to avoid contradicting them and causing further distress, so if they are recalling past events as if they are in the present, do not correct them. Instead, ask questions about their thoughts and keep them grounded in that time period without confusing them.

Compassionate communication is vital regardless of the stage of dementia. Ensure your loved one is comfortable and in a familiar, distraction-free environment. Be an attentive listener, paying attention to their words and emotions while maintaining eye contact and nodding to show you're listening. Don't interrupt them, even if they struggle to find a word. Show empathy through facial expressions and wait for them to finish their thoughts. When you have the chance to speak, use a friendly tone of voice and ask open-ended questions one at a time, giving them enough time to think and respond. If they do not hear or understand you, try rephrasing the question or repeating it in a different way. If they get frustrated, be prepared to change the subject or adapt your question to help them stay calm and comfortable.

When communicating, it is important to use simple and clear language, break down complex ideas into smaller parts, and speak slowly. This will help them follow your train of thought without confusion and give them time to process the information. You can also use gestures and facial expressions to convey your point. Your body language should be relaxed to help them feel more comfortable and supported. You can gently touch their arms or shoulders, or hold their hands to provide that extra comfort.

When communicating, it is essential to be sensitive and understanding. Therefore, there are certain things that you should avoid saying to them.

- **"Don't you remember this?"** This statement conveys frustration on your behalf and implies forgetfulness and can cause sadness and guilt.

- **"I just told you."** Communicating with someone with dementia takes patience. Repeat yourself calmly to help them understand, even if you just said something.
- **"You don't make sense."** They may feel embarrassed and ashamed that they're not communicating properly, even though they're trying their best. Instead, try to interpret what they said and repeat it back to them to confirm if you've understood their message correctly.
- **"You're confused."** It can be dismissive and embarrassing to tell someone "You're confused." Your family member may be confused, or they may have tried their best to recall a word and still ended up with the wrong one. Rather than writing them off, it's important to ask questions and try to understand what they meant.
- **"You should try harder."** It's important to understand that when cognitive abilities decline, it is crucial to support them in their efforts. This can be dismissive and may even discourage them from continuing to make an effort. This decline can be frustrating and can rob individuals of their uniqueness, so it's crucial to support them in their efforts. Therefore, it's essential to show empathy and support to help them through this difficult time.
- **"Don't be difficult."** It's important to avoid negative statements when communicating. Such

statements can escalate the situation and make them feel embarrassed or want to act out. Instead, it's essential to always remain patient and understanding. Remember that, although things may feel difficult for you, it's even more so for them.

- **"Do you remember who I am?"** Instead of asking this question introduce yourself by name and relation to avoid any confusion.
- **"Think harder so you can remember."** It's essential to understand that dementia and forgetfulness are not due to a lack of effort. Telling them to think harder so they can remember might not be helpful. They may already be trying their best, and pushing them to do more could make them feel like they're failing. This may discourage them from communicating altogether.
- **"You're making that up."** People with dementia can experience delusions and hallucinations, which may cause them to hear or see things that are not present to us. However, this doesn't mean that they're lying or making anything up. They could be sharing memories or feeling confused about the present moment, making it seem like they're imagining things. To ensure effective communication, validating their perceptions and asking questions is crucial. This can help make them feel comfortable and understood.

What You Don't Say Matters

Clarifying nonverbal communication is as crucial as choosing the right words when communicating.

Nonverbal communication is conveying messages without using spoken or written words. You can express yourself through body language, gestures, facial expressions, touch, eye contact, and posture. Even when communicating verbally, your tone, emotions, attitudes, and intentions come through your words. Thus, nonverbal communication complements verbal communication, making it more effective and impactful.

As a caregiver, understanding the different types of nonverbal communication can help you use them effectively.

- **Facial expressions:** Facial expressions are a powerful tool for conveying emotions. They can express happiness, sadness, rage, surprise, and terror. Common facial expressions include smiles, frowns, raised brows, and squinting. The more familiar you are with your family member, the easier it becomes to recognize and understand their facial expressions, drawing from shared experiences and memories.
- **Body language:** Body language pertains to the movements and postures of the body, such as slouching, crossing arms, nodding, and leaning in.

These signs can indicate curiosity, openness, defensiveness, or discomfort. However, many people are unaware of their body language when speaking, so it may take some time to consciously modify your body language to effectively communicate nonverbally.

- **Gestures:** Hand and arm movements known as gestures are used to communicate. Common gestures include waving, pointing, thumbs up, and making a peace sign. As cultures interpret gestures differently, it is essential to consider the cultural context one is drawing from and use them accordingly. You can also create custom gestures by showing and explaining what they represent. Use it as much as possible, and observe if they start to pick it up. You can invent gestures from scratch or use sign language as a starting point.
- **Eye contact:** Maintaining eye contact is a powerful nonverbal communication that can convey curiosity, attentiveness, trustworthiness, or intimidation. It's essential to note that the duration and intensity of eye contact may vary according to cultural norms and the interaction context. Therefore, it's crucial to be mindful of this fact to avoid making your loved one uncomfortable. Additionally, it's crucial to consider how much emotion people convey through their eyes. If you're feeling frustrated or

sad, they can easily pick up on that, and it could impact their mood. Therefore, it's best to try and remain upbeat when possible.
- **Posture:** How you sit or stand can reveal a lot about your attitude and mood. Standing tall and upright can show confidence while hunching over can show uncertainty. It's crucial to be aware of your posture when communicating nonverbally, especially since it can give away your emotions. For instance, if you're feeling tired, sad, or discouraged, you might unknowingly hunch your shoulders and your loved one may sense that. Likewise, when standing over someone who's seated, it's important to be mindful of your posture so that you don't come across as intimidating.
- **Touch:** Physical touch can convey a wide range of emotions and intentions, from tenderness and comfort to aggressiveness and boundary-setting. It can be an effective way to express empathy and support, especially towards older adults who often become socially isolated and do not experience the hugs and touches of friendship that younger people do. Gentle touching, giving hugs, and conveying comfort and security with your hands can help them feel connected to you and to society, thus enhancing their well-being.
- **Tone of voice:** As a caregiver, it's important to remember that nonverbal communication can still

include speaking aloud even if your loved one is unable to respond. Narrating what you're doing and explaining why can help with understanding. For instance, if they need to take a new medication with food, you can explain what you're doing as you prepare the meal. When speaking, use a calm, low tone of voice. Speak clearly, but avoid sounding like you're yelling or lecturing. Remember that voice tone, pitch, and intonation can all transmit emotions and attitudes. A soothing and warm tone may indicate, while a strong or loud tone may indicate irritation or anger. Stay aware of your voice as you speak.

- **Proximity:** During an engagement, the space between people can communicate comfort or discomfort. It is important to understand personal space norms that differ among cultures for effective communication. Since you share a past with your family member, you probably know if they prefer to be touched or keep a personal bubble. They may want you to sit next to them on the couch and hold their hand, or they may prefer you to sit in a chair nearby so they can have their space but still see you. Also, consider proximity in relation to your communication. If you are too far away, they may not be able to see you clearly.

Nonverbal communication is of utmost importance when you are taking care of someone, even if the person can still communicate verbally. A gentle touch can convey a lot of information, so be mindful of this while integrating nonverbal expressions into the process of caregiving.

This type of communication can be especially helpful when language skills decline. It can become quite challenging for them express themselves. In such situations, making eye contact, gently touching their shoulder, and giving them a warm smile can go a long way in showing how much you care, conveying empathy, and helping them feel connected to reality. This, in turn, strengthens your emotional connection with them.

Cognitive decline can cause agitation and anxiety due to confusion about their surroundings. Nonverbal cues such as gentle touches can help them feel more comfortable and secure, allowing them to stay calm. Providing reassurance helps them understand simple communication like gestures and basic sentences, without being distracted by confusion.

When communicating verbally is not possible, using nonverbal methods shows respect and dignity. Rather than talking for them or staying silent, this approach fosters a positive environment, encouraging them to feel safe and comfortable. By demonstrating this mode of communication, they will feel empowered to use it themselves, which can promote independence. They will be able to express their needs and desires through gestures, nods, and headshakes, and you will understand them better.

Nonverbal communication can be a powerful tool for monitoring the well-being of your loved one. You can observe physical discomfort or pain by paying attention to their facial expressions and movements. For instance, if they are limping or rubbing a shoulder, it may indicate they are experiencing some form of discomfort, even if they are unable to communicate it verbally.

In addition to facial expressions and touch, there are other methods of nonverbal communication that can help you stay connected, especially when they lose their ability to speak.

- When communicating with someone who has dementia, nonverbal cues are crucial. Make sure to maintain eye contact, nod your head to show that you understand, and lean in to indicate active participation in the conversation. Use nonverbal cues to validate the person's emotions and experiences. If they display despair or dissatisfaction, empathize with them by offering a reassuring touch or a compassionate facial expression.
- To effectively communicate information or instructions, use clear and simple gestures such as pointing and giving directions.

- Visual aids such as photos, charts, or written notes are extremely helpful in conveying information or reminders. They are particularly useful for keeping track of daily routines, prescription schedules, and identifying objects. It is advisable to incorporate personal objects or props that are relevant to the conversation or have personal significance as they can help to stimulate memory and communication.
- Match your emotional condition and demeanor to theirs. If they're nervous, be calm. If they're happy, express joy.
- Express emotions and connect through music, art, or other creative ways. These can be used to express feelings and connect with the person in new ways.

It's essential to pay attention to their nonverbal signals and adjust your communication style accordingly. If they seem upset or distressed, try different techniques to calm them down. Remember that every person is unique, and what works for one person may not work for another. When using nonverbal communication techniques in dementia care, it's essential to be flexible, patient, and empathetic. Focus on creating a caring and compassionate environment that fosters understanding and comfort, and follow their lead as much as possible.

The Art of Patience

Caregiving can be a challenging and demanding task, which can cause you to experience feelings of annoyance, discomfort, and even anger. These emotions are natural and expected, given the weight of your responsibilities. However, it's important to remember that reacting harshly or badly towards the person you care for can damage your relationship. Being patient with yourself and with them can help you stay calm and focused, and provide the best quality care possible.

Patience is a key factor in efficient communication in all aspects of life, especially when dealing with challenging or sensitive situations. Trust is the foundation of any relationship, and patience plays a crucial role in building that trust. Communicating patiently demonstrates your willingness to listen, understand, and value the other person's perspective. This trust is the cornerstone of open and honest communication and is an essential aspect of active listening, wherein you focus on the speaker without interrupting or rushing them. Patiently listening to someone encourages them to express themselves fully, resulting in more meaningful and effective communication.

Many issues and themes are complex and require time for people to express their thoughts and feelings. Patience allows you to manage these situations, giving the speaker space they need to express themselves fully. Patience is closely linked to empathy and compassion, enabling you to connect with others' emotions and experiences and demonstrate concern for their well-being. As a result, a helpful and caring environment is created. Patience is particularly crucial in caregiving roles such as healthcare or eldercare, where patient communication can reduce tension and worry and provide empathetic and respectful support to patients and clients experiencing physical or emotional difficulties.

Effective communication is a skill that involves understanding and adapting to the unique communication styles, speeds, and preferences of different individuals. Patience is a crucial aspect of effective communication, as it helps you to navigate these differences. Rushed or hasty communication can often lead to misunderstandings, misinterpretations, and conflict. Patience allows you to take the time to clarify information, seek clarification from others when necessary, and handle any doubts before they escalate into major issues. In situations where disagreements or disputes arise, patience is vital. It lets you remain calm and composed, even when emotions run high. This emotional stability enables constructive problem-solving and helps to establish common ground between individuals.

As a caregiver, you may often find yourself in situations where you feel helpless about your loved one's medical condition and their challenges. However, you have significant control over your emotional response to these difficulties, especially regarding negative emotions such as frustration and anger. Given the amount of effort you put into caregiving, you're likely to feel exhausted and stressed, which makes reacting impulsively appear to be the easiest option. However, practicing patience can help you to pause before reacting and respond calmly and compassionately to their needs.

Patience may not come naturally to everyone, but it is a skill that can be developed over time. It involves training yourself to remain calm, composed, and empathetic even in the face of adversity. There are several techniques you can use to cultivate patience, such as mindfulness, deep breathing, and cognitive reframing. By practicing these techniques, you can learn to manage your emotions better and respond to your loved one's needs with patience and kindness.

- **Self-awareness:** Start by identifying the situations or behaviors that tend to make you feel annoyed or angry. This way, you can recognize your triggers and learn to deal with those feelings in a constructive way. By identifying these triggers, you will become more self-aware and learn to manage your feelings with more patience
- **Mindfulness:** Stressful situations can often make it difficult to stay calm and respond appropriately. However, practicing mindfulness techniques such as meditation, deep breathing, and yoga can help you stay centered and minimize tension. One

helpful technique to calm down before responding is the 4-7-8 breathing method. In this technique, you inhale through your nose while counting to four, hold your breath for seven beats, and exhale through your mouth while counting to eight. Counting distracts your mind and slows your desire to respond immediately, giving you a chance to think calmly and react in an appropriate manner.

- **Communication:** Effective communication is essential during the caretaking process. It is crucial to be transparent and honest instead of hiding your true feelings behind politeness. This can lead to resentment building up and negatively impacting your relationship. When you feel resentful, it becomes difficult to show patience. Therefore, it is important to be kind in your tone and approach, but your honesty will help them understand your point of view. This way, you can work together to alleviate frustration. Of course, you should talk, but you should also be able to share your thoughts and experiences with others. This goes hand-in-hand with the next way to establish patience.
- **Support:** It can be beneficial to speak with others who are in a similar situation to yours because it can help you feel understood and improve your level of patience. By joining a support group, you can communicate with people who are going

through the same thing as you and receive feedback that can validate your emotions. Additionally, you can seek help and support from your friends and family members to assist you with your caretaking responsibilities or simply take a break from the routine and enjoy some socializing and fun.

- **Time management:** Effective time management can help you organize your caregiving responsibilities in a way that minimizes stress and helps you become more patient while carrying out tasks. Begin by scheduling all the necessary medical appointments in a calendar on your phone or planner. Then, include mealtimes and medication schedules to ensure that you are on track. Take time out for fun activities, such as listening to music or solving puzzles together. You can also plan community outings to keep your loved one engaged with the world around them. By visualizing everything on a schedule, you can feel more prepared and know what to expect.

4

MORE THAN JUST DAILY ACTIVITIES

There's a lot of power in our words, and there's a lot of power in our presence. You never know when that moment of connection can happen.

— RUFUS TONY SPANN

Thinking about time management is the perfect way to address the next aspect of the CARE+ model: activities. Daily care activities for people with dementia are essential for satisfying basic physical requirements and preserving general well-being by providing cognitive stimulation, involvement, and a feeling of purpose. These activities have a substantial impact on the overall quality of life.

THE CARE+ MODEL: ACTIVITIES

There will be many activities that you'll need to manage. Establishing a routine that gives them a sense of structure and predictability is essential. Consistency in activities can help reduce anxiety and disorientation by making their surroundings more familiar and comfortable. Routine tasks such as folding laundry, setting the table, and arranging personal objects can stimulate cognitive performance and help retain cognitive skills such as memory, problem-solving, and concentration.

Daily care activities can help maintain emotional connections and social interaction. Caregivers can encourage this by engaging in conversation, offering praise and reassurance, and promoting a sense of belonging and security. Performing daily chores to the best of their abilities can foster a sense of autonomy and self-worth, even if assistance is needed. By involving them in decision-making processes, such as choosing their clothing, they may feel empowered.

Creative activities like painting, drawing, and crafts can provide individuals with dementia with a way to express themselves and communicate, even if their speech abilities are limited. Listening to music or participating in reminiscing activities, such as looking at old photos or sharing stories, can evoke happy memories and emotions. Music is especially powerful in influencing mood and cognitive stimulation. Sensory exercises, such as touching different textures, smelling familiar aromas, or listening to natural sounds, can be relaxing and enjoyable. They can also trigger sensory memories and associations.

Participating in meaningful everyday activities can give people a sense of purpose and accomplishment while also improving self-esteem and overall well-being. Daily care activities go beyond functional chores, as they can stimulate cognitive function, create participation, and instill a sense of purpose. In addition, regular participation in daily care activities can help reduce challenging behaviors, such as agitation, anger, or wandering.

Caregivers, family members, and healthcare professionals should work together to plan and adjust daily care activities to the individual's abilities and preferences, resulting in a more meaningful and rewarding daily life.

Creating a routine that fits your loved one's lifestyle can make it feel like a natural addition to their day. To tailor it to their needs, consider their preferences and schedules. For instance, if they are not a morning person, schedule medical appointments in the afternoon instead of early in the morning. Observe when they appear most mentally alert and willing to go out or perform certain activities, and use that as the basis for creating a schedule.

Prior to planning any outings or tasks, take into account their health and medical requirements. If they have difficulty walking, an activity that necessitates walking may not be ideal. Always keep the medication schedule in mind so that you can provide them with the necessary medication at the appropriate times. In addition, think about their cognitive abilities and plan activities that appeal to them. For example, they may be unable to read the plaques in a museum, but they can still enjoy seeing the objects on display. They may appreciate the sensory experiences provided by children's museums, which allow them to interact with tactile exhibits. They may desire to visit a movie theater or prefer to sit in a quiet park to get some fresh air.

When planning activities, it is important to strike a balance between social outings and daily living activities. It's important to prioritize hygiene, nutrition, exercise, medical needs, and rest before scheduling any extracurricular activities. While educational outings are great, don't forget about activities that provide social interaction with others. Community centers and local libraries often host group activities that can be perfect for this. If they have friends nearby, try to schedule weekly or monthly meals or coffee dates with them.

In addition to socialization, it's also important to think about cognitive stimulation. Activities like memory games, playing cards, completing puzzles, reading, or engaging in hobbies are all great for boosting cognitive function and can be added to the routine. This downtime can provide relaxation while also reaping the benefits of cognitive stimulation.

In order to create an effective routine, it is important to incorporate variety. You should include a mix of necessary tasks as well as fun activities to prevent boredom and monotony. A well-rounded schedule that focuses on physical, mental, emotional, and social well-being should be provided. Having several activities in mind can also help with flexibility, as there may be situations where you need to cancel an activity or cut an outing short. Being able to adapt easily and knowing that there will be another opportunity to try the routine can help you adjust the schedule and keep your loved one happy and comfortable.

Apart from focusing on hygiene, mental stimulation, outings, and socialization, sleep is also a crucial factor in a quality routine. Many people with dementia experience insomnia or have difficulty staying asleep, so prioritizing sleep and being flexible may be your main concerns. If your loved one is too tired to go out as planned, you should let them nap as needed. Additionally, you should consider their sleep patterns when scheduling nighttime or morning activities. Give them enough time to wind down at night to prepare for sleep and just as much time to wake up in the morning before they start their day.

When going about your daily activities, it is crucial to prioritize safety. Take the time to research the places you plan to visit and ensure that the environment is free from any obstacles that could lead to accidents. Make proactive arrangements for modifications and accommodations like a scooter or elevator access.

It is equally important to schedule downtime for yourself in your routine. Your well-being is just as important, so it's essential to avoid burnout. If you're not in a good place yourself, you cannot help anyone else. Therefore, take time to relax, socialize, and indulge in your hobbies.

Keeping a schedule can be helpful in managing your time effectively. You can either keep a mental note of the routine or have it written down. One useful tool is to use your phone calendar as it can be synced with your computer and give alerts, reminders and alarms. For those who prefer paper plans, consider color coding appointments to easily see what's on for the week at a glance. It's also beneficial to keep records of your activities to track what you've done and how well it worked. Adding notes, including the reactions, will help you plan later outings. It can also help you gradually introduce new things. By looking back at your schedule, you can see that you went on an outing last week that seemed overwhelming, so you can wait to schedule another instead of demanding too much too quickly. Additionally, you can involve them in the process as much as possible. Working together can help them understand what's to come in the next few days so they feel more independent rather than feeling like you're doing everything for them.

Sample Daily Care Plan

It is important to create a daily care plan that provides structure and support while addressing their individual needs and abilities. To do this, you should consider their preferences, routines, and cognitive abilities. An effective care plan should be structured into morning, afternoon, and evening phases. Here's an example of how to divide a daily care plan into these.

Morning

Starting the day at the same time every day can help establish a healthy routine. Assist them with their hygiene, such as washing their hands, brushing their teeth, and getting dressed, while encouraging them to do as much as they can independently to promote a sense of self-reliance. Adjust activities as necessary to ensure their safety and comfort. For example, they may require help holding the toothbrush, while they can still hold it, or they may need assistance getting dressed, in which case you can let them choose what to wear or provide them with options to participate in the decision-making process.

Make sure they have a nutritious breakfast that meets their dietary requirements and provides enough energy to last until lunchtime. Help them by cutting up food or feeding if necessary, but still encourage them to be independent. Instead of holding a spoon or fork in front of their face, ask if they're ready for another bite. If they can't verbally respond, you can develop a sign to ask if they're ready for more. Even holding up an empty utensil and raising your eyebrows can function as a question, and they can nod or shake their head in response. This seemingly small gesture empowers them to maintain control over their lives and demonstrates respect for their personhood, which is incredibly valuable.

After breakfast, they should be awake enough for some cognitive stimulation. You can show them photos, and let them reminisce or talk about current events if they are aware. You could also read to them or play a game, like cards or even Twenty Questions. It is important to choose activities that align with their interests and try to offer a new one every day. For example, you can do the same thing every Monday, but don't repeat it every other day of the week. To gain the full benefits, it would be helpful if you mixed up these activities.

Once they have exercised their mind, it's time to move their body. The physical activity should be light and customized to their abilities. You can do gentle stretches or take a walk, allowing them to set the pace and offering your arm if they need support. While you'll want to mix up their activities, you can do the same physical activity as often as necessary, especially if they're limited in their choices. It's more important to get them to move their body than it is to do something different each time.

After physical activity, ensure they take morning medications as required or necessary.

Afternoon

It is important to serve a balanced and nutritious lunch that will provide enough energy for the rest of the day. Since they may be excited about the morning's activities, it's best to sit with them and engage in conversation to help them stay calm and focused on the meal. Your loved one may feel eager to do more activities and try to rush through the meal, but it's crucial to give their body time to get the necessary fuel.

After lunch, it's essential to encourage rest and taking a break. They don't necessarily have to take a nap, but they should relax and engage in quiet activities like reading a book or listening to soft music to process the morning's activities. This rest, coupled with the nutritious lunch, will provide them with enough energy to get through the rest of the day.

Once they have had some quiet time, your loved one will likely be ready for social interaction. This is a great time to schedule visits with friends and family, talk on the phone, or participate in community programs or support groups. Socializing is essential for well-being and will help them feel connected to others.

Encourage them to engage in a creative activity while riding on the excitement of socializing. If they already have a hobby they enjoy, such as painting, support them in doing what they already know. However, if they are not artistic, don't skip this part of the routine as they may still enjoy attempting to paint, draw, or color. Their mind is different now, and they may connect with this activity. Crafts are also a great option as they involve the practical and creative parts of the brain, as well as hand-eye coordination. If they are unable to do the creative activity on their own, you can adapt it for them. For instance, you could help them paint by gently enclosing your hand over theirs on the paintbrush. Hold it up to the canvas and let them guide you slightly to create the design, allowing them to feel creative and independent because they were part of the process.

After completing the activity, it's a good idea to enjoy a healthy snack together. This will keep them on a balanced diet without ruining dinner. Pair the snack with water to keep them hydrated.

Evening

When planning evening activities, it's essential to consider sundowning. Many people tend to get more confused later in the day, so it's best to avoid scheduling major activities. Instead, try to keep evenings relaxed and low-key to promote reasonable bedtimes and healthy sleep.

It's a good idea to involve them in dinner preparation, but safety must be a top priority. If it's not safe, you can start making dinner while they're eating a snack so that you're in the same room with them and can keep them involved in the process from a distance. Even if they can't help with cooking, they can bring you ingredients and be a taste tester. Remember to make dinner nutritious and filling, and sit with them at the table to encourage them to take their time eating for better digestion.

Like after lunch, the post-dinner lull is a great relaxing time. This will help them feel sleepy and ready for bed. You can encourage them to read, listen to music, or watch a TV show, but it's important to turn off all screen usage about an hour before bed to ensure they don't stay up too late.

Establishing a comforting bedtime routine is a great way to help with relaxation and prepare for sleep. You can assist with tasks such as bathing, brushing their teeth, using the bathroom, and changing into pajamas. Take your time and create a calm environment to help them feel sleepy. Make the routine enjoyable so they look forward to it and don't resist sleep. If they need medication, be sure to give it to them before leading them to their bedroom. You can read to them or talk quietly, but make sure the topics are neutral to avoid agitation and difficulty falling asleep.

Remember that the above daily schedule is just a suggestion; you can modify it to fit your needs. Flexibility and adaptation are key when caring for someone with dementia. Be open to changing your daily care plan if their requirements or preferences change. Regularly assess and communicate to ensure their comfort and well-being. If possible, involve additional caregivers and family members to provide support and respite, so you can maintain your overall well-being.

Personal Care: Bathing, Dressing, Grooming

Taking care of daily activities like bathing, clothing, and grooming is crucial to ensure that your loved one stays clean, comfortable, and healthy. These activities also play a vital role in preventing physical health concerns, such as skin disorders or infections, which are common in dementia patients. As dementia progresses, your family member may find it more challenging to take care of themselves. With impaired memory, they may forget the steps of washing and dressing or how to use soap and water effectively. They may also skip essential steps in brushing their teeth and putting their shoes on before clothing.

Dementia can also affect spatial awareness, making it difficult to maneuver around small bathrooms, judge the distance to the toilet or sink, and use razors or toothbrushes properly. This can lead to safety concerns, such as forgetting to turn off the water, using extremely hot water, or falling over while getting dressed or cleaned.

It can be challenging to help with dressing and maintaining their hygiene. Their bladder and bowel control loss can make the process even more complicated. You might have to start all over again after helping them bathe and dress due to an accident. Communication issues may also arise, making it difficult for them to express their needs. Thus, you have to be patient and attentive.

Your loved one may feel agitated during the process, as they may not want your help or feel uncomfortable with anyone in their personal space. Therefore, you should approach them with care and ensure that they feel comfortable. It is essential to show them that you want to help them complete tasks rather than take over their independence.

Before helping with bathing and dressing, you should understand the challenges involved. You should assess their abilities and allow them to be as independent as possible while monitoring their condition. You can also seek guidance from their medical team to understand what tasks you need to take on.

When providing care, personalizing your approach is crucial. Even if you get information from a book, a medical professional, or a support group, you know them better than anyone else. You understand the type of touch that comforts them and what might make them uncomfortable. Always respect their preferences and boundaries, provide them with privacy when possible, and encourage them to care for themselves as much as possible.

Allow ample time for each task to promote independence for as long as possible. Be patient and give enough time to do things at their own pace. This may require you to adjust your daily schedule, but it will help them remain calm and confident in their ability to care for themselves.

When you need to assist them, engage them in the process by asking questions like, "Would you prefer a shower or a bath today?" This gives them a choice while emphasizing that this step is essential for their hygiene. Praise them for doing something independently or helping you, as positive reinforcement can be beneficial. Keep your instructions clear and concise, as you do with all your communication, to avoid confusion or forgetting tasks.

It is important to prepare the space in advance, whether you are in the bathroom or bedroom. Ensure the room is well-lit and free of obstacles that can cause tripping. If they are taking a bath or shower, ensure the water temperature is neither too cold nor too hot. Keep everything they need within reach, such as soap, towels, and fresh clothes. It may also be helpful to create a visual chart that outlines the steps involved. If you are able to, create a large numbered list with pictures of the shower running, using soap, rinsing off with a cloth, drying off with a towel, and getting dressed.

It's important to remember that a bath or shower isn't always necessary. You can use washcloths or baby wipes to stay clean every other day or two between showers. They will feel fresh and clean without undergoing the lengthy process of a bath or shower. This can be particularly helpful if they are resistant to bathing.

Some individuals may have difficulty changing their clothes. If their clothes are not dirty, you do not need to help them change daily, as long as it does not affect their health and well-being. However, if it does, you should let them choose their clothing from a few comfortable options. If they do not like you assisting them with dressing up, consider using elastic waistbands and shirts that button up in the front so they can pull everything on and do it themselves. Distracting them by engaging in a conversation may also help.

It can be helpful to involve your them in every step of the process when it comes to picking out clothes. Start by going clothes shopping together and help them find things that are comfortable, easy to put on and fit them well. Let them choose the colors and patterns they like the most. You also need to consider their sensory preferences, such as whether they prefer soft fabrics with no scratchy tags or long sleeves instead of short. Once you find something they like and can put on independently, consider buying the same garment in different colors to make the process even simpler. Following the daily routine mentioned in the previous section can significantly help in combating any challenges.

Having a daily routine can be very helpful in combating resistance when it comes to bathing, cleaning or changing clothes. By establishing a routine, they will know what to expect and when to expect it, which may make them more willing to participate without experiencing agitation.

However, if you continue to experience issues, you may want to consider altering the routine to a more suitable time of day.

Oral Hygiene and Toileting

Maintaining good oral hygiene is essential for keeping the mouth healthy and free from pain. Daily tooth care is an essential part of their hygiene routine and can help prevent various dental issues in the future. You may need to use adaptive tools like toothbrushes with larger handles or electric toothbrushes to make the process easier for them. Supervising them initially is also important to ensure they do it correctly. If they can do it independently, let them continue until you notice any change in their oral hygiene or abilities.

As dementia progresses, you may need to brush their teeth for them. Using a soft toothbrush is best to avoid applying too much pressure. Alternatively, you can use disposable foam swabs to clean their teeth and gums without worrying about bristles. Please make sure they're comfortable and relaxed while cleaning their teeth. Consider using distractions like quiet music or talking to them. Don't forget to keep up with their dentist appointments to monitor their oral health.

Using visual charts can be incredibly helpful for maintaining hygiene. You can put a chart next to the sink that shows the toothpaste going on the toothbrush first, then brushing teeth, rinsing the brush, and putting it away.

This will make them feel more independent and less reliant on assistance.

It is essential to take good care of the teeth, as it can prevent serious dental problems. However, even with proper care, there is still a chance that they can develop gum disease or tooth decay. Regular dental checkups can help detect these issues early on, and the dentist can provide the necessary treatment. In the case of periodontal disease, it is important to treat the gums gently to avoid any irritation. This includes flossing, which can be challenging, but must be done. Tooth decay can be caused by diet, so it is crucial to monitor the consumption of sugary snacks and drinks. Regular brushing, mouthwash, staying hydrated, and taking fluoride supplements can also help prevent tooth decay.

In case there is loss of some or all teeth, dentures may be a suitable option. Dentures can help them chew properly and improve their appearance. However, there is an adjustment period, during which they may find it challenging to speak or eat normally due to the unfamiliar teeth in their mouth. With practice, they will learn to adapt. It is recommended that they sleep without their dentures, which will require cleaning with a brush and denture cleaner.

As time passes, the mouth may change, and they may require new dentures. The dentures may also break or get lost, so it is essential to ensure they fit securely and have a designated location for storage and cleaning to eliminate the risk of losing or breaking them.

Maintaining oral hygiene is considered personal, as it requires putting your hands in or near someone's mouth. However, if you are a caregiver, you may need to assist with toileting, which is also a sensitive process. In such a scenario, it's crucial to exercise patience and understanding while promoting dignity and privacy to ensure everyone's safety and calmness.

Having a set bathroom routine can make the process easier and more predictable. Encourage them to go to the bathroom when they wake up, after meals, before leaving the house, and before bed. You can add additional instances when you notice them needing it. While having a routine won't prevent all accidents, it can be helpful. If they resist using the bathroom or say they don't need to, gently prompt them without giving them a choice. You can say, "It's time to use the toilet now." This phrase sounds agreeable and may encourage them to try even if they don't think they need it. You can further help by providing step-by-step instructions such as "Let's go to the bathroom," "Sit down on the toilet," and "Wipe yourself clean." You may require assistance in undressing, getting them in a comfortable position, and wiping them. If you're worried about their privacy or dignity, you can cover them with a towel or clothing to help everyone feel comfortable.

It is important to prepare for accidents when dealing with incontinence. You can identify triggers that cause loss of control, such as certain foods or activities, and work around them by scheduling bathroom breaks or using absorbent pads or adult diapers. These products can provide comfort in emergency situations and prevent embarrassment after an accident.

Privacy is crucial for your loved one's dignity. You don't want to be overbearing, which can lead to frustration and mistakes. To promote bathroom independence, ensure that the bathroom is safe by installing handrails and raised toilets. Use low mats with non-slip backing to prevent tripping and ensure proper lighting to help them navigate and access toiletry items such as toilet paper and soap.

Nutrition, Hydration, and Medication Management

Maintaining a healthy diet and staying hydrated are crucial for overall physical and mental well-being. Meal preparation and eating together can encourage optimal nutrition and hydration while providing sensory stimulation through taste, smell, and texture, making it a fun and engaging activity. You can involve them in meal planning to an extent they feel included, and when you offer healthy options, they're empowered to make good choices and influence their diet and nutrition.

However, individuals with dementia may struggle with eating proper meals due to forgetfulness, changes in taste and smell, or difficulty swallowing. Dental issues that interfere with chewing and side effects from medication can also make mealtimes more stressful. Despite these obstacles, a balanced diet rich in essential nutrients, vitamins, and minerals can support brain function, promote healthy bone growth, and provide enough energy to get through the day. Adequate nutrition can help retain muscle mass and maintain an ideal body weight.

While that information sounds very straightforward, the issue with dementia patients is that they may be too forgetful of eating, experiencing changes in taste and smell, or struggle to swallow. These obstacles make the seemingly simple tasks of eating proper meals seem more daunting and frustrating. When you add dental issues interfering with chewing and possible side effects from medication, mealtimes can become very stressful.

Having regular meals scheduled is vital to supporting nutritional needs. Offering delicious food they enjoy is crucial in promoting a healthy appetite. Still, to balance it with healthy options or limit intake of less-healthy favorite foods. Ensure they have plenty of water during the meal and stay hydrated by drinking water, juice or eating fruit.

It's possible that your loved one may not be getting all the nutrients they need from food. If this is the case, talking to their doctor about adding supplements can help ensure they get the vitamins and minerals necessary for optimal health.

As dementia progresses, eating habits may change. It's important to be flexible and ensure that you give them healthy food they like, regardless of their preferences and routines. What they once enjoyed may not taste the same anymore, so don't make them feel bad for this change or force them to eat it. Mealtimes should always be calm, with no need to rush, which can cause safety issues regarding chewing and swallowing or make them feel like they don't have enough time to eat all they want. You may find more minor, frequent meals appealing instead of three larger meals daily.

Dementia can affect coordination, leading to difficulty in holding utensils. In such cases, you can consider using adaptive utensils, such as weighted spoons and forks, to help balance food and feed themselves. Finger foods can also be a good option, as they are easier to grasp and eat independently. However, they may struggle with chewing and swallowing as the condition progresses. In such cases, softer or pureed foods can be helpful, and you can consult a dietitian for texture-modified diets.

A high-fiber diet may avoid constipation. Serve fruits, vegetables, whole grains, and plenty of water. Constipation can cause discomfort and negatively impact their health, so being proactive with their nutrition is essential.

In addition to a well-balanced diet, taking medications as prescribed is equally important. Following the prescribed medication regimen is essential to maintain health and well-being. You may need to keep their medication locked away to prevent them from taking it themselves. Although it's great to encourage independence, they may forget that they've already taken a dose and take another, which can be harmful to their health. By overseeing their medication dosage, you're keeping them safe.

To ensure you don't forget refills, organize medication in a pill dispenser or organizer. An established, consistent routine can help eliminate any mistakes regarding medications. You can use a calendar or create a medication chart and mark off each dose when given. This way, you can keep track of everything and avoid any confusion.

Certain medications may worsen symptoms of dementia. Consulting with your doctor is important and having knowledge of potential medication side effects will enable you to act as an advocate at the doctor's office.

Anticholinergic medicines inhibit the function of the neurotransmitter acetylcholine and are used to treat a number of illnesses, such as allergies, gastrointestinal issues, and Parkinson's disease. Diphenhydramine (Benadryl) and oxybutynin (Ditropan) are two common examples. Side effects include dry mouth, constipation, blurred vision, increased heart rate, and cognitive impairment.

Benzodiazepines are central nervous system depressants that are often given for anxiety, sleeplessness, and muscle spasms. Diazepam (Valium) and alprazolam (Xanax) are two examples. Side effects include drowsiness, memory issues, risk of falls, and a dependence on the medication that can cause withdrawals in the long run (Lundberg, 2023).

Corticosteroids, which include prednisone and dexamethasone, are anti-inflammatory drugs used to treat a variety of illnesses, such as autoimmune disorders, allergies, and asthma. Side effects include suppressing the immune system, osteoporosis, mood swings, elevated blood pressure, and gastric irritation.

Beta-blockers such as metoprolol and atenolol are used to treat high blood pressure and heart disease, whereas statins such as atorvastatin and simvastatin are used to decrease cholesterol levels. They can slow the heart rate, decrease energy levels, cause dizziness, and reduce blood flow to extremities. Muscle pain, liver enzyme elevation, and gastrointestinal symptoms are also commoFgiletten.

Chemotherapy drugs are another type of medication that doesn't work well for dementia patients. They cause fatigue, nausea, vomiting, mouth sores, bone marrow suppression, and cognitive changes. When paired with dementia, these medications can have a major detrimental effect on the mind, including more memory issues and trouble focusing (Gillette, 2023).

Promoting Physical Activity

Regular physical activity, which may include activities such as stretching, walking or simple exercises, can help maintain physical health and mobility. Participating in these activities releases endorphins which can improve mood and reduce agitation. Depending on the condition of their dementia, there are different activities that both of you can do together. However, before incorporating any physical activity into their daily routine, it is essential to consult with their medical team to ensure the activities are safe for them.

Incorporating physical activity into the routine has a multitude of benefits. Although it will not slow the progression of the condition, it can significantly enhance the quality of life, improve memory, and help them learn new information. It can also lead to an improvement in concentration and decision-making abilities. Regular physical activity can also boost mood, improve sleep quality, and reduce feelings of agitation and restlessness. Additionally, exercise can improve their physical health, help maintain strength and mobility, and prevent falls and fractures. It can also help in weight management, improve circulation, and promote heart health.

If you go on walks, you both can enjoy the benefits of exercise. If they attend a physical activity class for senior citizens, you can take some time off while also being assured that they're safely engaged in exercise.

However, before you encourage them to engage in any physical activity, it's important to consider their preferences and abilities. You want to choose activities that they enjoy so that they'll be motivated to participate. Additionally, when they feel capable, they'll experience a mental health boost that will make them feel independent. While the primary focus of physical activity is on the body, it's also important to encourage sensory stimulation by adding music, games, and aromatherapy to the mix. Engage their mind with different textures, colors, sounds, scents, and tastes to make the experience more enjoyable.

When engaging in activities, it's important to incorporate familiar things that can trigger memory. This can be things from their past or repeating activities they are already familiar with. Consistency and repetition can help them feel safe and supported. Even when repeating an activity, it's essential to provide clear and simple instructions or visual cues to help them feel confident in themselves. Uncertainty can cause mood swings or lead to losing balance and falling, so clear guidance is crucial.

Consider ensuring that physical activity takes place outside. They can enjoy nature and get fresh air, boosting their mood and overall sense of well-being.

While it's important to balance physical activity with rest for optimal health, you need to take time to rest, as you'll learn in the next chapter.

Share the CARE+!

It is not the load that breaks you down. It's the way you carry it.

— LENA HORNE

We talk about 'emotional rollercoasters' all the time, but, in my experience at least, there's no situation where the expression fits better than caring for a loved one with dementia.

As they lose more of the person they once were, you find yourself grieving for that person at the same time as managing their often challenging behavior and savoring the moments of lucidity during which you can bond. You might feel the full gamut of emotions within the space of an hour.

I think this is one of the most exhausting parts of caring for someone with dementia, and the CARE+ model is a way to make it more manageable because it incorporates you as the caregiver as well as the needs of your loved one.

A holistic approach is really the only way to tackle dementia because it affects every single angle of daily life. Taking care of yourself has to be a part of that because it's the only way you can show up, consistently bringing your best.

But unfortunately, there are far too many caregivers out there suffering in silence and struggling to meet their own needs as they look after their loved one. I wanted to share the CARE+ model to try to counteract this, and although I know you have many demands on your time right now, I'd like to ask for your support in reaching more carers.

By leaving a review of this book on Amazon, you'll show other people caring for a loved one with dementia where they can find the guidance they so desperately need.

They're looking for this information, and your review will help them find it quickly – and it won't take long for you to leave it either.

Thank you so much for your support. I know you understand how important this is.

Scan the QR code below

5

RESTING YOUR HEART

Self-compassion is simply giving the same kindness to ourselves that we would give to others.

— CHRISTOPHER GERMER

Caring is more intense and a full-time job because the work never stops. You, your family, or nurses are on the clock day and night, ensuring your loved one is safe, calm, and looked after. However, it's a balancing act, because you still want to treat them with respect and dignity. It's also more involved than a job because of the close relationship. It can feel impossible to untangle yourself from caregiving to take a break. Unfortunately, if you don't prioritize your own rest and resilience, you can't be an effective caregiver. That's what the CARE+ model focuses on: your rest and resilience.

THE CARE+ MODEL: REST AND RESILIENCE

When you're a caregiver for a loved one, you prioritize their well-being above all. Many people who care for family members with dementia think that they need to give their all since they can't do much for themselves. They feel like they can give 110% of themselves for as long as needed, then catch up on rest and self-care when the loved one is in a nursing home, hospice, or someone else's care. However, pushing yourself too hard and waiting for relief leads to burnout, which is detrimental to both you and your family member.

Your schedule is busy when you're caring for someone else, but if you establish a schedule as previously recommended in this book, you should be able to free up some time for yourself. If you push away the feelings of guilt that prevent you from indulging in self-care, you'll feel much freer about the opportunity. Instead of thinking that you're spoiling yourself with self-care, maybe frame it as self-neglect when you're putting everyone else's needs above your own. You deserve care and free time just as much as everyone you're helping, so there shouldn't be any guilt.

Barriers to self-care may also include finances, exhaustion, and a mounting list of responsibilities. However, remember that self-care doesn't have to cost money, and it doesn't need to involve you going somewhere. You can take advantage of your usual evening downtime to do something at home for yourself, like eating your favorite meal while you binge-watch your favorite show. Or even allow yourself to fall asleep on the couch while reading a book. The freedom of doing what you want and not feeling like you need to stick to your strict routine of being in bed by a certain time can help you feel more relaxed and indulgent, which will prime you to give better caregiving the next day.

Care for the Caregiver

Though it may feel strange to prioritize yourself, start with small goals that don't require much effort. For example, instead of booking a spa day, make time to take a hot shower or bath that can ease your sore muscles. Choose things that genuinely sound restful to you so you enjoy doing them instead of feeling obligated to mark "self-care" off your to-do list. It may help to mention your intentions to a friend or family member so they can ensure you take this time for yourself and hold you accountable.

Caregiver burnout is a state of physical, emotional, and mental tiredness experienced by people who offer long-term care and support to those who are ill, incapacitated, or otherwise unable to care for themselves. Caregivers frequently endure a high level of stress and responsibility in their roles, which can lead to burnout if not appropriately managed. This experience is the result of the emotional and mental strain, physical exhaustion, lack of personal time, and financial strain. Caregivers can also struggle with role confusion, because they must balance between acting like a family member and nurse in all situations.

If you're feeling burnt out, you should try to arrange respite care. Even a temporary break from caregiving can give you time to relax and feel more like yourself again. If family members or friends offer to help, take them up on it, even if you don't typically accept help. Planning ahead in terms of extra help and financial issues can feel like a light at the end of the tunnel and help lessen the stress that leads to burnout.

One of the easiest ways to give yourself time off is to prioritize your sleep. Aim to get at least seven hours of sleep each night. You can create a calming bedtime routine of disconnecting from screens, listening to quiet music in a dimly lit room, and bathing or handling skincare to encourage yourself to fall asleep easily and improve your sleep quality.

Another way to care for yourself while you're a caregiver is by eating healthy meals and exercising. Since your loved one also needs these benefits, you should eat meals and exercise right along with them. You'll get time together but still be fueling your body with the vitamins and energy it needs.

Whenever you're stressed or have downtime, mindfulness, meditation, and breathing exercises can help you relax quickly. I mentioned the 4-7-8 breathing method in Chapter 3 regarding patience, but it helps here as well. Just as that exercise is short, making just a few minutes for meditation can make you feel relaxed and destressed, like a mini-break from your caregiving duties.

Caregivers have limited leisure time, so these high-impact self-care activities will take you 10 minutes or less. You don't need to carve out a portion of your day for self-care; simply remember these tips and use them as needed.

- **Deep breathing exercises (2 to 5 minutes):** Find a quiet place, sit comfortably, and focus on your breath for a few minutes. Inhale deeply for four counts, hold for four counts, and exhale for four counts. Repeat multiple times to help you relax and reduce stress.
- **Short break (2 to 5 minutes):** Pause and be totally present in the situation. Close your eyes, take a few deep breaths, and look around you without judgment. This can assist in resetting your perspective and reducing stress.
- **Mini meditation (5 minutes or less):** To quickly calm your mind and relieve tension, use a meditation app or a brief guided meditation video. There are numerous apps that provide brief

meditation sessions that are adapted to busy schedules.

- **Stretching (2 to 5 minutes):** Stretching can help you relax and enhance your circulation. Stand up, extend your arms overhead, touch your toes, or do some fast neck and shoulder stretches.
- **Affirmations for success (1 to 2 minutes):** To improve your attitude and self-esteem, repeat a positive statement. Start with phrases like "I'm doing my best" or "I am strong and resilient."
- **Play uplifting music (5 minutes or less):** Put on your favorite song or playlist that elevates your spirits and enjoy it for a few moments. Music has an instant and positive effect on your mood.
- **Visualization (5 minutes or less):** Close your eyes and imagine a quiet and serene area, such as a beach or a forest. Focus on the peaceful sensations and noises in your head as you imagine yourself there.
- **Tea time (5 minutes or less):** Make a cup of your favorite herbal tea and sit down for a few minutes to enjoy it. The warmth and aroma can be soothing and pleasant.
- **Practice gratitude (2 to 3 minutes):** Make a list of three things you're thankful for. Practicing thankfulness can help you focus on the positive aspects of your life and improve your attitude.

Sitting With Complex Emotions

As mentioned in Chapter 2, caregivers experience complex emotions during this time. Sitting with your feelings can help you accept them and understand what you're going through without feeling overwhelmed by stress.

The first step is to recognize your feelings without judgment. You don't need to understand why you feel a certain way, just name it. For example, you may think, "I'm sad," or "I'm frustrated." That's all you need to do initially because it's accepting your emotions without suppressing or denying them.

Next, understand that you'll feel both positive and negative emotions in your life. There's no way to ensure you're always positive, and though you may worry that you're always negative, that's not the case. Things look different when you're stuck in them, so knowing that you'll experience both can help you feel more neutral about where you are right now.

While you sit with your emotions, breathe deeply, emptying your lungs and pulling in fresh air with each breath. This process will help you stay present without allowing your emotions to overwhelm you. It also helps you observe your emotions without attachment. You'll feel less tempted to deny, suppress, or change them. You'll understand that they're temporary and will flow throughout the day, so there's no need to cling to them or assign them too much importance.

Making time to assess your emotions will help you practice self-compassion. Treat yourself as you'd treat a friend. That means you're not beating yourself up over anything you feel, but rather acknowledging it and striving to express it in a healthy way. Healthy outlets for emotions include talking to friends, family members, or therapists. You can also use creative approaches like journaling, drawing, painting, or listening to music.

Balancing Caregiving and Personal Life

The best way to balance caregiving and your personal life is to set clear boundaries between the two. It is important to create a comprehensive schedule and adhere to it as closely as possible. That may mean asking other people to take on certain shifts so you can go to work, spend time with family and friends, or just take time for yourself.

Prioritizing your tasks can also help you achieve this balance. Start by analyzing your personal life and identifying what matters the most to you. If you have limited spare time, think about how you would like to spend it. What would you do if you had more free time? What would you do if you had a day off? By evaluating your responsibilities and hobbies, you can manage your time effectively and ensure that you have enough time for both enjoyment and relaxation. Also, consider delegating some of your tasks to others. For instance, grocery and meal delivery can be a great option if it's difficult to get away from home. By outsourcing some of these chores, you can free up more time for other important tasks.

It can be difficult to take on this major caregiving role in addition to your regular life, so try to balance them by first being honest with yourself. You know how much you can handle, so don't push yourself to take on too much and think you'll pull it off somehow. You're capable of a lot in life, but caregiving is very difficult, and you shouldn't feel guilty about setting limits in terms of how you can help.

If you have a job, look into your benefits. You might be able to establish your loved one as a dependent and help them with some of your services. You may also have the ability to take time off to care for them without losing your job. Depending on your career, you may want to talk to your direct report about working remotely or making your job more accessible so you can still be a team player at work while being a caregiver.

Things don't always work out the way we want them, though, so it's best to have a backup plan. Consider who else can share some responsibilities while you work and manage your personal life. Look into adult day care options or see if you can afford an in-home nurse. Social services can help you find quality nurses and nursing homes, plus assist you in obtaining funding as well.

Building Resilience

The ability to bounce back from adversity, obstacles, or tough experiences and adapt effectively to life's setbacks is resilience. It's the ability to tolerate and recover from stress, trauma, or hardship in order to regain mental, emotional, and physical well-being. Resilience is more than just surviving problems; it's also about thriving in the face of them.

Resilience includes adaptability, emotional regulation, and problem-solving skills. People who are resilient have a positive outlook and continually learn from their experiences to become better. However, resilience isn't an inherent trait; it can be developed over time. When you're caregiving, resilience is a crucial characteristic.

Building resilience is a dynamic process that entails cultivating psychological and emotional strengths in order to effectively deal with adversity and recover from failures. Start by cultivating a positive mindset. This can be difficult when witnessing suffering, but expressing gratitude for the opportunity to care and spend time with them can help develop a positive attitude. Embracing change and flexibility is crucial for resilience and positivity. Relying too heavily on one thing can lead to difficulties if things don't go as planned. A resilient person, however, can adapt to new circumstances and find alternative solutions without getting too discouraged by setbacks.

Resilience requires self-care and emotional regulation. If you let your feelings take over, it's going to feel too challenging to bounce back. Sitting with your emotions, as previously discussed, can help you accept them and let them go. It's a form of self-care that helps you build your confidence and feel more comfortable in who you are. This confidence, along with your sense of purpose as a caregiver, can give you the push you need to overcome challenges and build your resilience.

Lean on Support Groups

Caregiver support groups are useful places for people who are caregivers to share their experiences, seek advice, and be encouraged. These organizations foster a supportive environment in which caregivers, regardless of their situation, may learn from one another's experiences and collaborate to overcome common issues.

Whether you're caring for a family member at home, dealing with the complications of Alzheimer's disease or other kinds of dementia, or managing care in a care facility, the collective expertise within these support groups is a great resource. Participants in these groups might have a fresh perspective and unique solutions to comparable caregiving issues by learning from the varied array of experiences shared by their peers.

Caregiver support groups, in essence, promote an environment of shared knowledge, empathy, and mutual aid, where the difficulties of caregiving are alleviated by the power of collective wisdom and compassionate support.

When dementia is diagnosed, the doctor may give you information about local support groups and other resources. This is a great place to start reaching out. You can also look at the Alzheimer's Association online map to find support groups in your area. AARP and the Parkinson's Foundation also have information about community-based support groups (Ghebrai, 2021).

If you're unable to find a support group in person, you can also find this type of community online. There are many private Facebook groups, like the Dementia Caregivers Support Group, Alzheimer's and Dementia Caregivers Support Chat Group, and the Caregiver Support Community. Private groups allow you to open up and share your experience honestly with only other approved members. You can join by signing in to Facebook and requesting to join a private group. They may ask questions to verify you're a person instead of a bot before acceptance. If you're not on Facebook, you can also get help on AgingCare's Caregiver Forum.

HOME, SWEET HOME

Home isn't where you're from; it's where you find light when all grows dark.

— PIERCE BROWN

The ability to take care of your loved one in their home is a major benefit. You don't have to worry about uprooting them and sending them to an impersonal nursing home at a time when they need a lot of support and compassion. However, you need to ensure their home is a safe place for them where they can be comfortable and independent for as long as possible.

THE CARE+ MODEL: ENVIRONMENT

Dementia impairs the mind in many ways and can make a home unsafe. Even if they've lived in the same place for many years, the condition changes judgment, depth perception, sense of time and place, and behavior. These changes can create a perfect storm, leading to confusion and instability. The tips in this chapter will help you keep their home a safe, comfortable place to stay and remain independent as long as possible. In addition to modifications, providing close supervision during cognitive changes can enable them to stay in their preferred environment.

Ensuring Safety in the Home

Dementia has a significant impact on safety in multiple ways. Behavioral changes can manifest as heightened agitation and aggressiveness, leading to less calm and collected reactions than before. If they get angry and confront someone, they may fall or have an accident. Additionally, they become more forgetful, increasing the chances of leaving the oven on, forgetting to lock the doors, or wandering outside at night.

Your loved one's body is aging as their mind changes due to dementia. They're not as strong as before, so they may have issues with balance, coordination, and mobility. They might start shuffling their feet to walk instead of picking them up, tripping easily over carpets. They can get up too quickly and become dizzy and disoriented, causing a fall. Dementia can also affect the senses of the affected person, leading to changes in vision and hearing. Poor vision can cause them to not notice obstacles in the way as they are walking. If they have auditory issues, they may not hear instructions or warnings as they are on the move.

You can ensure safety in the home by making thoughtful modifications to what's already there. Check all the light fixtures in the house and ensure they have bright bulbs to illuminate all areas of the home. Shadows can cause confusion as they walk around, while bright lights will keep their vision as clear as possible. You may also want to add night lights in hallways, bedrooms, bathrooms, and the kitchen, so they have automatic lights if they get up in the night. Motion-activated lights are ideal as they turn on automatically.

Check all furniture in the home and think critically about what is essential. Keep their favorite and most comfortable couches and armchairs, but if the living room is cluttered, eliminate unnecessary furniture to keep open spaces and clear pathways. Replace some of the soft chairs for more supportive models with sturdy armrests that make it easier to stand up. Consider upholstery that's easy to clean in case of any accidents.

Flooring can have a significant impact your loved one's safety. If there are any loose, decorative rugs, move them into storage to eliminate the risk of tripping. You may want to consider removing wall-to-wall carpet and install wood or nonslip flooring to provide additional security and avoid potential accidents. Ensuring the color of the floor contrasts with the walls to improve depth perception. This will make them more surefooted and comfortable when they need to put their hands on the wall for support.

Safety in All Areas

Bright lights in the kitchen and dining areas ensure visibility while eating and drinking. Use colorful tableware so they can tell the difference between the plate and the food on it. Plates with compartments may help them scoop up food more easily without pushing it onto the tabletop. Adaptive utensils will also help them stay more independent in terms of feeding themselves.

The bathroom has many safety risks, so ensure it is well-lit and has nonslip mats on the floor and in the bathtub. Installing grab bars in the tub and near the toilet can help maintain balance and comfort. It will also give them something to pull up on so they can stay independent with bathing and toileting.

Labeling items in all rooms of the house can significantly enhance independence and safety. For example, in the bathroom, keep toothpaste handy and clearly labeled, while keeping the medical ointment tucked out of the way to prevent confusion. Ensure your loved one knows where things are placed. Involve them in the organization process and arrange things in logical places so they can locate what they need. Beyond labeling each item, you can also label drawers, cabinet doors, and storage containers with words or pictures so they know what's inside. This will also prevent them from rummaging around and losing items or encountering dangerous objects when they're feeling restless as they will know exactly what's inside a drawer or cabinet.

However, access to everything is not necessary. You can install locks on certain cabinets that contain chemicals in the kitchen and bathroom and install safety knobs on the stove. There are also knob protectors for doors that will ensure they can't lock themselves out of a room.

In addition to standard safety concerns around the home, you should also think of major events, like a house fire. Install smoke detectors in bedrooms and hallways, testing them regularly and replacing batteries as needed to ensure they will function in case of a fire. Keep fire extinguishers in accessible locations, typically the kitchen or garage. Develop a fire escape plan they can remember and practice it often. Remind them about several possible exit options in case one or more are blocked by fire. Establish a safe meeting point away from home, but close enough to prevent them from getting lost.

With that in mind, you will also want to address wandering. People with dementia often have trouble sleeping and get up to wander the house because they feel restless. However, this puts them in danger because they're walking in the dark and may even attempt to leave their home. To combat this, you can install motion-activated night-lights to provide illumination. Door alarms can alert you when the door opens so you know when their headed outside. Setting up a safe outdoor area is ideal so they can get fresh air without leaving the property. Consider fencing in the yard or creating a small, enclosed patio to give them this option. You'll want to ensure they always have identification with contact information on them so someone can help them reach you if they get lost. The most effective method for preventing wandering is through proper supervision.

Creating Comfortable Spaces

Creating comfortable living space at home can help alleviate the agitation caused by dementia. When surrounded by familiar items, they feel more calm and secure, which can combat agitation that may lead to frustration, anger, insomnia, and wandering. While you should keep the space as clean as possible with plenty of room for accessible mobility, there's nothing wrong with keeping loved furniture and displaying their favorite decor on the walls to help them feel connected to their past. They'll have a greater chance of remembering things from their personal history and will feel more in control of their home, ultimately giving them confidence in their actions.

Reducing clutter is key for comfortable spaces. That doesn't mean you have to get rid of everything, but only keep what's necessary. Once you have the items they want or need to keep, carefully organize and store them in a way that is easy to find, but does not create clutter in walking or sitting areas. In fact, instead of putting photos, travel souvenirs, or heirlooms in storage, you may want to find ways to display them on the wall or mounted shelves so they can see them and feel inspired to remember those times.

It's important to create quiet spaces, even if they enjoy watching TV or having background noise. You can set up comfortable chairs where they can sit to read or listen to music, or designate a specific spot at a table or use a TV tray so they can enjoy puzzles or games without being distracted by the TV or other noises.

While providing care, it is important to create a calming environment that stimulates their senses. Soft, neutral colors are best for walls, decor, and furniture because they're not so vivid that they'll cause overstimulation. Consider adding blankets in neutral colors as well, selecting various textures to further engage the senses. Natural lighting is ideal during the day as it can naturally encourage sleep patterns by allowing plenty of sunlight during the daytime. Use curtains or blinds to control the light in case it's too bright. You can also bring nature inside by growing plants in pots around the home.

Choose a mix of flowering plants in different colors and greenery that they can smell and touch.

Maintaining Independence for as Long as Possible

Caring for someone with dementia is challenging, especially when they are used to living independently. They may feel like they are being treated like a child, which can be frustrating for them. It's essential to keep them as independent as possible to help them feel like themselves, which can reduce their stress levels and keep them in good spirits. You can achieve this by providing them with adaptive aids and tools that offer assistance while maintaining their dignity, respect, and privacy. Prioritizing independence not only enhances their quality of life but also reduces the caregiver's burden as the loved one feels empowered to do more for themselves.

Memory aids are one of the most effective tools to prolong independence. This includes digital reminders and voice-activated assistants, such as Amazon's Alexa. This technology can be used by asking it to turn on lights, change the temperature, set reminders and alarms, and add items to a grocery list without relying too much on memory. Medication dispensers with alarms can also be a reminder when it's time to take their pills. Additionally, using the calendar functions on phones, tablets, and computers can help them stick to a schedule without needing constant reminders.

Making the house a safe environment will also boost their independence. Reduce the risk of falls by eliminating rugs and carpet, adding nonslip mats in the kitchen and bathrooms. Grab bars are great for assistance in the bathroom, near the toilet, and in the bathtub, but you can also install them in hallways and on the stairs to give your loved one something secure to hold onto as they walk around. A personal emergency response system is another assistive device worth looking into. Necklaces, bracelets, and pins with a call-for-help feature are also available. There are also wall-mounted alarms you can install around the house.

Creating an Engaging Home

Since you're making the home such a comfortable place to be, make their time even more enjoyable by offering engaging activities they can participate in without leaving the house. While you want them to get out in the community and socialize whenever possible, having activities ready at home for days when they don't feel like going out ensures they don't miss out on crucial cognitive activity.

Expertise is not required to enjoy time together doing any of the activities listed below. Sometimes, trying something new can activate different parts of the brain and create a sense of inspiration. These activities are just starting points, so you can use them to get started and then add more activities based on how well they respond to them.

Arts and Crafts

- Create greeting cards to send to family and friends.
- Use magazines, photographs, and colored paper to create collages.
- Paint with watercolors using large brushes with grips.

Music and Singing

- Listen to music they love or songs from their childhood.
- Sing along with their favorite songs.
- Play musical instruments like bells, tambourines, and shakers to keep the beat.

Memory Games

- Play matching games with cards that have big pictures and bright colors.
- Look at photo albums and ask questions about what's happening in the pictures.
- Play "I Spy" games using things you see around the home.

Gardening and Nature Activities

- Planting and watering flowers in a garden or inside.
- Arranging flowers in a vase for indoor enjoyment.
- Birdwatching or looking for animals through the windows or on short walks.

Baking and Cooking

- Working together to follow a recipe and make a meal or dessert.
- Choosing recipes that work well to make a delicious meal.
- Helping in the kitchen by mixing, stirring, or decorating the final project.

Puzzles and Games

- Piece together jigsaw puzzles with large pieces.
- Play games like Bingo, Checkers, or Memory.
- Enjoy card games with simple rules like Crazy Eights, Solitaire, and Go Fish.

Storytelling and Writing

- Tell stories from their past inspired by their memory or photos.

- Write short notes and cards to send to family and friends.
- Working together to compile a journal or scrapbook of thoughts and memories.

Physical Activities

- Go for short walks around the block or in the yard.
- Dance to their favorite songs.
- Slow-paced exercises like chair yoga and stretching.

Sensory Activities

- Spend time with touch-and-feel books or sensory boards to feel unique textures.
- Massage their hands and arms with scented oil or lotion.
- Taste different foods to enjoy distinct flavors and textures.

While you may enjoy doing these activities together, you can also harness the power of technology to give them the chance to exercise their mind more independently. Tablet and smartphone apps can help boost their brainpower and memory. Look for games like Sudoku and crossword puzzles. There are even app versions of coloring book pages that allow them to create beautiful images by tapping the color and the correct part of the page to "color" it digitally. There are apps and websites like Lumosity, Elevate, and Peak that offer more complex brain training programs. These programs require daily effort to help improve brain power gradually over time. You can set an alarm to remind them to complete the exercises at the same time every day.

You can also introduce technology to offer access to new activities. One great example is a virtual museum visit. Many world-famous museums have this option on their website. You can also find similar videos on YouTube.

Virtual pet sites and apps can be a great option for someone who loves animals but cannot take care of a pet or have a dog or cat at home. These platforms can provide a way to feel the joy of caring for a loving companion without the added responsibility of another life to take care of.

Tailoring activities to your loved one's interests, abilities, and stage of dementia is the key to successful involvement. To ensure that these activities are fun and meaningful for the person with dementia, stay flexible and patient and create a calm, supportive environment. Involving family members and friends in these activities can also promote social interaction and create memorable moments together.

INTERACTIVE ELEMENT: HOME SAFETY CHECKLIST

Follow this checklist to ensure you're keeping the home as safe and comfortable as possible.

- Store medication, alcohol, matches, knives, tools, and cleaning products in cabinets with locks to prevent accidental use or ingestion. Have the number for poison control saved in your phone or posted on the refrigerator.
- Install smoke and carbon monoxide detectors and check them often, including changing the battery as needed.
- Keep walkways clear of rugs and clutter and ensure they're well-lit to prevent tripping.
- Ensure chairs are comfortable, sturdy, and have supportive armrests.
- Secure large furniture like TVs, shelves, and cabinets to the wall so they won't tip over.
- Remove locks from interior doors or install special knobs that prevent them from locking themselves in or out of a room.
- Add stove knob covers to prevent accidental turning on or leaving on.
- Install grab bars near the toilet and bathtub in the bathroom and possibly along the walls in the hallway and on the stairs.

- Put nonslip mats on the kitchen and bathroom floors and in the bathtub.
- Lower the maximum temperature on the water heater to prevent scalding.
- Installing a home security system can help you stay informed and alert you immediately of any opened doorways.
- Subscribe to a personal emergency response system so they have a button on their person or in the house to quickly and easily call for help.

7

FOR YOUR PEACE OF MIND

Planning is bringing the future into the present so that you can do something about it now.

— ADAM LAKEIN

So far, the bulk of this book has addressed hands-on care issues, as that's what most people think when caring for someone with dementia. When you're struggling to keep your loved one calm, comfortable, and healthy each day, it's hard to pull back and see the bigger picture—but it's necessary. That's why part of the + in the CARE+ model covers the legal and financial considerations you'll eventually encounter.

THE CARE+ MODEL: LEGAL AND FINANCIAL CONSIDERATIONS

Legal and financial issues for someone with dementia are critical in order to preserve their well-being and protect their rights as their cognitive abilities deteriorate. These factors include a variety of legal documents, financial planning, and decision-making processes. As their caregiver, you'll want to ensure they have everything in place to protect them as their cognitive abilities decline.

Important Legal Documents for Dementia Care

Legal documents are extremely important because in safeguarding the rights and decision-making independence of people living with dementia. These essential legal documents allow pre-designated individuals to make decisions when they are no longer able to do so. Specific legislation and procedures governing these documents may vary depending on your jurisdiction.

Standard Will

A will is a legal document outlining a person's wishes regarding how their affairs are managed and assets distributed after their death. It's the most common estate planning document, so if one doesn't already exist, get one written before it's too late. Doing so when they're still of clear mind will ensure their wishes are followed and legal issues are prevented.

Wills include asset distribution that explains how someone's property, money, investment, and possessions should be split between their beneficiaries. Since beneficiaries can include family members, friends, charities, and other entities, having everything detailed in a legal document is crucial.

The will can also establish an executor. This is the person who will carry out the guidelines listed in the will, including managing the estate, paying debts, and distributing the remaining assets according to the will. Debts and taxes must be settled first and the executor will oversee this prior to distributing the remaining assets to beneficiaries.

If case anything isn't mentioned in the will, it's automatically part of the residual clause. This specifies how assets or property should be distributed to beneficiaries. This ensures that if a valuable item is not included in the will, it will be part of the residual clause.

In addition to financial matters, the will can also include information about funeral and burial wishes. They may specify their preference for burial or cremation and the location for their remains.

If a will hasn't been created, you can help them think about what they want to include. However, in most places, they'll need to consult a lawyer to create a legally binding document. There may also be a requirement for witnesses and a notary to validate the will. It is important to note that a will is an amendable document which can be modified.

While a basic will is an important estate planning document, it may not cover all elements of someone's financial and legal concerns. Additional estate planning tools, such as trusts, advance directives, and beneficiary designations, may be recommended to handle more complex or unique needs, depending on one's specific circumstances.

Consulting with an estate planning attorney can assist in creating a well-crafted, basic will that appropriately reflects their wishes and complies with local laws and regulations. Furthermore, estate planning can assist with minimizing tax costs, protecting assets, and ensuring that their legacy is managed in accordance with their wishes.

Additional Legal Documents

Additional legal documents such as advance directives, powers of attorney, and guardianship are essential instruments for ensuring that the preferences and interests of individuals with dementia are honored even as their cognitive competence declines. These documents allow the appointment of trusted individuals, usually family members or close friends, to act as advocates and decision-makers when they are unable to articulate their preferences or make informed decisions due to the progression of dementia.

Living Wills and Advance Directives

Living wills or advance directives establish healthcare choices including decisions on life-sustaining therapies, resuscitation, and end-of-life care. These documents provide guidelines for medical personnel and family members to ensure that their healthcare decisions are consistent with their previously expressed preferences.

Power of Attorney

Power of attorney (POA) delegates legal authority to a trustworthy person to make financial and legal choices on behalf of the person with dementia. This covers financial asset management, bill payment and execute legal documents. The POA safeguards financial security and guarantees that their commitments are met.

There is also a POA for healthcare, called a Healthcare Proxy or Medical Power of Attorney. This can allow a trusted caregiver or family member to make their healthcare decisions when they're unable to. They can also communicate with healthcare providers and understand the complexities of the persons medical records and treatment options, assisting them in making informed decisions.

Guardianship and Conservatorship

Guardianship or conservatorship may be undertaken as a more complete legal alternative when a person with dementia is no longer capable of making decisions in their best interests and other legal documents are not adequate. The court appoints a legal guardian to make decisions about personal care, medical treatment, and financial affairs. This procedure entails a thorough examination of the person's capacity and is often used when no other options are available.

Living Trust or Revocable Trust

A living trust or revocable trust gives your loved one the opportunity to place assets in a trust while they can still make choices, designating one trusted person to manage assets for distribution to the beneficiaries. This can avoid probate court in case the person with dementia becomes incapacitated or passes away.

Physician Orders for Life-Sustaining Treatment

Physician Orders for Life-Sustaining Treatment (POLST) or Portable Medical Orders are issued by healthcare providers based on the patient's preferences and previous wishes regarding medical interventions. The medical team will consider the intensity of potential treatments and the frailty of the patient to understand if the treatment is beneficial considering the advancement of their condition. Filling out a POLST form necessitates a conversation between the patient, their healthcare professional, and, in some cases, their family or healthcare proxy. This dialogue ensures that the patient's values, goals, and medical state are considered while writing the orders. In POLST, the term "portable" alludes to the document's ability to go with the patient across various healthcare settings. It's usually printed on bright, clearly identifiable paper, such as pink or orange, to stand out in medical records. A POLST can be prepared in addition to other legal documents. POLST is best appropriate for those who have significant, life-limiting illnesses or are nearing the end of their lives. It's especially important for those with advanced dementia, whose healthcare preferences may change over time as the disease develops.

These legal agreements have distinct functions and are vital instruments for people to plan for financial, legal, and healthcare requirements, particularly in cases of incapacity caused by dementia. Because the specific regulations and requirements for these contracts differ by jurisdiction, contact legal practitioners who specialize in elder law or estate planning to ensure that these forms are correctly executed and in accordance with applicable laws.

Handling Legal Paperwork

Ideally, basic legal documents are already in place and if aren't, you should help them file these as soon as possible. This will ensure they are thinking logically and are aware of the boundaries they're establishing regarding their care and assets. You can periodically review the paperwork with them and ensure it aligns with their wishes.

Although it's difficult to think about these things, having these documents on file now will greatly streamline the process when your loved one passes away. You'll will most likely be overcome with grief, so eliminating the need to spend time consulting with lawyers and going to court will only benefit you in the long run.

Even with legal documents on record, you'll still need to obtain death certificates to confirm the death with legal entities such as corporations and insurance providers, in order to close out all existing accounts. Contact banks, credit card companies, investment firms, and the Social Security Administration. Also reach out to government organizations such as the Department of Motor Vehicles, property assessor, and municipal utilities. Check accounts that may be on autopay and cancel those payments and send the death certificate to those companies to close the accounts. Document the entire process, as dealing with such a major loss can be overwhelming and you may need proof of the steps you have already taken.

Financial Planning for Long-Term Care

While the legal paperwork described above can put their affairs in order, the financial side of things is much different. Many people can live a long life, even with dementia, so you should consider the costs of nurses or nursing homes.

Caregiving can be a costly affair, even though you may not receive any payment for your time and effort. You may have to bear the expenses of their rent or mortgage, utilities, phone, TV and other services such as their personal emergency response or home security system. If they still have a car, you may also have to pay for their registration, insurance, and gas if either of you still drives. To save money for future care, it's worth examining the current expenses and finding ways to cut costs.

Assessing current finances involves reviewing their income, assets, debts, and expenses to clearly understand how much money they must rely on for future care. Use this information to create a long-term care budget, but also be aware that insurance, Medicare, and Medicaid may provide some support.

You also need to research in-home dementia care and other costs you may encounter. Factors will vary depending on your location, the degree of care you need to provide, and how long you'll have to provide it while giving up other aspects of your life. As previously discussed, you should also consider what modifications you need to make to the home and property to prioritize safety and comfort. You might change the decor, buy more supportive furniture, repaint the walls, and pull up the carpet to prevent fall risks on the floor. Grab bars, security systems, and ramps are other costs you may encounter.

Caring for someone with dementia most likely will involve medical expenses. You may need to pay for medication and possibly cover copays for medical appointments. Additional assistance may also be required, such as a hospital bed, oxygen, or a nurse. Depending on the availability of help, you might have to allocate funds to pay for a nurse when you're unavailable or when you need some time away. While certain insurance plans may cover some expenses, the overall costs of dementia care can quickly add up, reaching tens of thousands of dollars or more, depending on lifespan, the cost of living in your area, and medical needs.

Caregivers who need to restrict their work hours or leave their jobs entirely encounter even more financial issues. Providing caregiving may lead to significant expenses while having little or no income. While insurance may cover some medical costs, the cost of living can still add up and become a burden on everyone involved.

When estimating the costs associated with home safety, accessibility, and overall comfort, it's important to factor in various expenses. This includes checking prescriptions and insurance policies to determine any out-of-pocket costs for doctor visits and medication purchases. Additionally, mortgage or rent payments, bills, and groceries should be considered. As a caregiver, it's important to set aside money for temporary nursing services to allow yourself a break. By estimating these costs upfront, you can prepare for potential long-term care facility expenses and assess what resources you have available.

When trying to understand their financial status, there are various documents you can refer to. Bank statements, property deeds, and insurance policies can provide insight into their savings, property value, and life insurance coverage. Additionally, they may have investments and retirement accounts from their employment, such as an IRA or a 401(k). If a will was created, it can be a valuable resource as it will outline their net worth and who they intend to leave their possessions to. By examining these documents, you can gain a better understand of their estate.

In addition to the financial documents, you should consider yours as well. This is especially true if you're taking a leave of absence from work and aren't making as much money as you typically do. You need to review your bank accounts and if you will have enough money to make ends meet while caregiving.

Having all the financial information available, you can create a budget that ensures your loved one and you can live comfortably without any financial stress. Establishing a certain level of financial security will greatly benefit both of you, as it alleviates stress and allows you to focus on caring and spending quality time with them while they are still lucid.

In your role as a caregiver, you may need to pay for various expenses while providing care. You might be eligible for certain tax benefits and deductions as a result of your caregiving responsibilities. You should also note that tax regulations can be intricate and subject to change.

Therefore, it's recommended to seek guidance from a tax professional or reach out to your local tax authorities for personalized advice that aligns with your specific circumstances.

Your tax benefits may include caregiver tax credits and deductions. They vary by state, so check your local laws. This federal tax credit will lower your tax. If you're paying someone to help with the caring, you may be eligible to claim the child and dependent care credit which may cover up to 35% of your care expenses.

It's important to plan ahead and budget for expenses in the year following passing.

If possible, you should consider meeting with a financial planner, lawyer, or social worker to understand the possible costs and available options for assistance. There may be government programs and community resources that, in addition to insurance, can alleviate the financial burden. If your loved one is a veteran, they may be eligible for certain benefits from the Veterans Administration (VA). The Aid and Attendance benefit compensates veterans and their spouses who require assistance with daily life activities due to dementia or other diseases. Medicaid is a government program that provides low-income people with healthcare coverage, including those who require memory care. State eligibility requirements and covered services differ. Some states provide waivers designed expressly for home and community-based memory care services.

Paying for memory care can be expensive, but there are several ways to finance it. Many people pay for memory care with personal savings, assets, and income. Creating a budget and a financial plan can help manage these expenses. Long-term care insurance policies may cover the costs of memory care services, depending on the policy's terms and the care required, so review the insurance policy to determine what is covered. Life insurance policies may provide alternatives for accessing the cash value of the policy or using accelerated death benefits to meet memory care costs. Consult with your insurance company to learn about your alternatives.

If benefits and savings have been exhausted, it might be time to consider a more serious approach to their finances. Some people utilize their home equity to pay for memory care. Reverse mortgages, home equity loans, and selling the home are all options for accessing the equity. However, it is important to make a detailed assessment of the impact on housing stability and financial security. Personal assets such as real estate, vehicles, and valuable items may also be sold or liquidated to cover memory care costs. Consultation with a financial expert can assist in determining the best course of action. While money for quality care is necessary, selling precious items can cause distress at a time when they are already easily agitated. Therefore, it is important to take these steps carefully and seriously consider the value of selling certain items compared to the emotional impact it may have.

KEY TIPS FOR DEMENTIA CAREGIVERS

- Create a financial plan and budget that allows funds for dementia care and potential emergencies.
- Establish a power of attorney for finances and a healthcare power of attorney for medical decisions. This can be the same person or different trusted individuals.
- Be cautious of scams and allowing interaction with people who are targeting them because of their mental state.
- Periodically review their financial plan and will to ensure they are updated if their needs change.
- Seek advice and feedback from dementia care organizations and support groups that can give you information you need from people who have gone through similar situations.

8

LOOKING AHEAD

The end of life deserves as much beauty, care, and respect as the beginning.

— ANONYMOUS

Once you have your finances in order, you want to look ahead to end-of-life care. This subject is a difficult one to think about, but knowing your options and having a plan in place can greatly streamline the process. Since you thought ahead, you're able to appreciate your time with your loved one even more, knowing they'll have the best care possible at the end of their life. Planning ahead also means you have the chance to make more thoughtful, compassionate decisions instead of feeling pressured to take immediate action before it's too late.

THE CARE+ MODEL: CARE OPTIONS AND END-OF-LIFE CARE

While you may appreciate being your loved one's caregiver and having the chance to bond, there may come a time when this isn't sustainable, or they need more assistance than you can give. With that in mind, you should know the care options, as they all offer various levels of support and may have expenses associated with them.

Exploring Care Options

Depending on your needs and preferences, there are various options for care available. You can use a combination of these options with your own caregiving, or you can opt for one of these entities to take full responsibility for the care of your family member.

In-Home Care

In-home care encompasses an array of caregiving options. You can hire nurses to help with medical needs or someone who can provide companionship. If you need assistance with bathing, dressing, and feeding your family member, you can get help with those services. They can provide regular shifts or offer relief to primary caregivers.

The best way to find in-home caregivers is to look at online directories, contact agencies, and get referrals from people with experience in dementia care. If you're part of a support group, you can ask for recommendations and use those as a starting point. Conduct your own research into the provider's credentials and ask for references and reviews. When selecting a care provider, it's essential to schedule an interview to ask questions about the specific care they provide, as well as the process of interaction. The costs of their services will vary depending on the type of services required.

Adult Day Care

Adult day care centers provide a chance to get out of the house and socialize with other people. These day care centers have activities, crafts, and field trips for dementia patients. Many also offer meals and therapies to attendees so they can get everything they need while you're at work or taking a break from caregiving.

Look for adult day care centers in your area and research their reputation and the services provided. Schedule a visit so you can tour the facility and meet the staff. Ask about their credentials and safety procedures. If specialized care is required, ensure that this facility can accommodate their needs before committing to service. Costs will vary depending on the facility and the services they offer, but many accept insurance or Medicaid.

Respite Care

Respite care is a flexible way to have short-term care at home or a facility. You can arrange to receive in-home respite care or a short-term residential stay while you tend to your mental or physical health, work, or family obligations. It's a great way to take a break from caregiving without compromising your quality of care.

It's normal to feel guilty or anxious about this option, but remember that it can be the best solution for everyone involved. Taking a break from each other can be beneficial for both of you. It can help you appreciate each other even more when you reunite. You'll have the opportunity to take care of your personal life while being confident quality care is still being received. Additionally, this cost might be covered by insurance or Medicaid.

Hospice Care Services

When a person is nearing the end of their life, Hospice care can provide comfort and quality of life. Hospice care is focused on meeting the emotional and physical needs of the individual rather than solely on medical treatment. If someone has a terminal diagnosis with a life expectancy of six months or less, they may be eligible for hospice care. Hospice providers are experienced in keeping patients comfortable during the final stages of their lives. If eligible, it may be possible to receive unlimited hospice care.

Hospice teams typically comprise doctors, nurses, counselors, and social workers, who work together to relieve pain and other related symptoms. They offer support to both the patient and their family, and you can work collaboratively with them to create a plan that meets your specific needs. Additionally, the plan can be tailored to include religious or spiritual aspects to help with end-of-life care and preparation.

Hospice care is available to dementia patients regardless of where they live, and can be provided in a variety of settings, such as their own home, a nursing home, a hospital, or a hospice center. Medicare, Medicaid, and many insurance plans cover hospice care, which can provide significant support to both the patient and caregivers.

Long-Term Care

Long-term care includes retirement homes, nursing homes, assisted living, memory care units, and life plan communities. If you can no longer provide care at home, consider long-term care facilities. These facilities provide a supervised location where their own space is available. Long-term care facilities have nurses, doctors, and staff to assist with daily tasks. These facilities offer meals, activities, and field trips for those who can participate. You can visit and take them out for the day or special events.

There are different levels of involvement in each facility, so it's crucial to explore your options and ask questions to ensure its the right fit. For instance, if your loved one is still active and independent, they wouldn't want to live in an assisted living facility; instead, a retirement home with scheduled events and outings may be a better option. Additionally, it's important to look for a facility that provides more care as their dementia condition changes. Lastly, consider the costs, as many facilities may not accept private insurance.

Regardless of the type of care you choose, there are some questions you'll want to ask as you interview staff and tour facilities.

- Find out if the home and caregivers are licensed and accredited according to state and national agencies to meet care standards.
- Inquire about the staff-to-resident ratio and on-staff medical personnel.
- Take a tour to assess facility safety for fall hazards and access. Inquire about emergency procedures and staff's ability to assist those with dementia.
- Ask about all services, included fees, and potential additional care as needed.
- If the patient desires to leave the facility for outings, ensure that the organization provides this service. Additionally, inquire about the in-house activities offered to stimulate mental activity.
- During your tour, observe the cleanliness and maintenance of the facility which can impact one's well-being.

- Ask about resident policies to understand room items and visitation.
- Always ask for a detailed breakdown of costs to avoid unexpected fees when making payments.

Making Decisions for End-Of-Life Care

When close to passing away, it's important to provide end-of-life care. This involves ensuring comfort and freedom from pain, allowing for a peaceful transition. Regardless of whether your loved one is suffering from complications due to dementia or old age, this is a difficult time, which is why it is crucial to prioritize their comfort and enhance their quality of life.

Planning for the decline in mental capacities due to dementia is crucial. When you plan, it can make this time easier for everyone involved. It is essential to discuss your loved one's wishes during this process, including their preferences for pain relief and emotional support. Doing so will allow them to pass with dignity and have a say in their care until the very end. Knowing that you are carrying out their wishes will give you peace of mind to help you through the grieving process.

When approaching the end of life, it becomes crucial to focus on managing physical symptoms, such as pain, discomfort, and agitation. Emotional support is equally important, and it's essential to consider the patient's and their family's psychological needs. It's necessary to respect and treat their wishes with dignity to ensure they receive the care they need and deserve. This approach can help reduce stress and grief for everyone involved. By providing comfort, you can focus on spending quality time with them while they are still with you, which can bring peace of mind to everyone.

End-of-life care often requires a team of professionals. You can include doctors and nurses to provide medication and pain relief. Hospice workers will coordinate care and provide emotional support for the patient and family. Social workers can help with emotional aspects and also help you navigate the next steps such as funeral plans, death certificates, and financial related matters. If you're spiritual or religious, you can bring in chaplains or spiritual advisors can be brought to provide assistance. Psychologists and counselors can also be included in the team to help everyone understand the end of your loved one's life.

During the late stage of dementia, it's essential to plan for end-of-life care. The late stage of dementia is characterized by severe memory loss, difficulty in communication, and the need for assistance with basic activities such as walking and sitting. The person may lose interest in their hobbies and experience weight loss and increased agitation due to difficulty eating. They may also have trouble sleeping and appear unaware of their surroundings. It's important to recognize the signs of this stage and begin planning for their care accordingly.

End-of-life care for a dementia patient should be personalized, compassionate care that prioritizes comfort and dignity. This involves continual communication and collaboration between healthcare providers, the patient, and their family to ensure that the individual's needs and wishes are met throughout this difficult period.

Discussing end-of-life care is crucial to ensure that appropriate care and support is given. Initiating these conversations as early as possible is advisable, allowing ample time to plan and make well-informed decisions regarding care goals and preferences. Look for opportunities to bring up the topic naturally and keep the conversations brief. Feeling anxious or apprehensive during these discussions is natural, so be kind to yourself and your loved one. Understanding their desires is important for their peace of mind. As you navigate this emotional journey, remember to take care of yourself by seeking the necessary support and resources to maintain your well-being.

If the necessary paperwork is not in place, the end-of-life process may look different. Medical choices are often made in accordance with the "best interests" standard. This implies that healthcare practitioners and, if required, the court will examine what is best for the person with dementia, taking into account their medical condition, values, and any information about their preferences that is accessible.

Healthcare providers often consult with family members to understand a person's preferences and values. While family members may offer suggestions, the healthcare team makes the final decision after consulting with ethical committees or other specialists.

When family members face disagreements or difficult decisions regarding medical care, legal action such as guardianship or conservatorship may be necessary.

It is important to note that the legal process and standards for decision-making on behalf of someone with dementia can vary significantly depending on the jurisdiction. To ensure that decisions are made in accordance with the law and in the best interests of the person, it is advisable to seek guidance from a local elder law or healthcare law attorney. Advance care planning, which includes preparing an advance directive, is highly recommended to specify preferences and select a trusted individual to make decisions when dementia or other conditions affect decision-making ability.

It is crucial to converse about end-of-life wishes while they are still mentally sound and lucid. Involving attorneys and judicial systems in such matters can be burdensome, so it is important to honor their wishes and prevent potential conflicts or stress. Even though it may be difficult to talk about such a sensitive topic with someone you love, it is important to make them a part of the decision-making process.

CONCLUSION

Caring for someone with dementia can be a challenging but deeply fulfilling journey that tests your tolerance, compassion, and resilience. It requires physical and mental strength and a comprehensive understanding of the unique needs and experiences of those affected by this condition.

As a caregiver, you provide unwavering compassion and care for someone who may not always acknowledge or remember your efforts. You witness the gradual decline of memories and abilities while providing comfort and companionship, ensuring every moment is dignified and respected.

In the face of the unrelenting growth of dementia, caregivers learn the importance of adaptability and ingenuity in finding new ways to communicate and interact with their loved ones. They become advocates, navigating the complex healthcare and legal systems to ensure they receive the best care and quality of life.

Along the way, caregivers may face frustration, loss, and tiredness, but they also discover a great power within themselves. Despite the difficulties, they find solace in the small, treasured moments of connection and delight that can still occur.

Caregiving is a testament to the power of love and the resilience of the human spirit. It is a role that demands self-care, support, and the willingness to seek help when needed. At the same time, it is a position that offers tremendous opportunities for personal growth and the chance to significantly impact the life of someone you care about and you will discover an inner strength you never knew existed. This newfound strength will give you the confidence to face any future obstacle that may come your way.

Taking care of someone with dementia can be an enduring act of love, but it's also a test of patience, courage, and resilience. Despite its ups and downs, caregiving allows individuals to offer comfort, dignity, and a long-lasting impact on the lives of those they care for. It's a journey that reminds us of the importance of empathy, compassion, and human connection.

As a caregiver, you encounter moments of strength and unconditional love. You discover opportunities to connect with your loved one on a deeper level, even in the face of dementia's challenges. You find strength in small pleasures, shared smiles, and warm embraces. Caregiving is a tribute to the ever-lasting power of compassion, and each day presents a chance to make a positive difference in the life of someone you cherish. Caregivers provide necessary support, and create a cocoon of love and understanding that envelops their loved ones, bringing brightness and meaning to each day.

Be the Guiding Light for Another Carer

As you know very well, people choose to care for their loved ones because they want to be there through all those moments... and as you also know, that isn't always easy. You can make the journey a little easier for someone else by leaving a review.

Simply by sharing your honest opinion of this book and a little about your own journey as a caregiver, you'll help other carers to find the help they're looking for.

IN UNDER 1 MINUTE
YOU CAN HELP OTHERS JUST
LIKE YOU BY LEAVING A REVIEW!

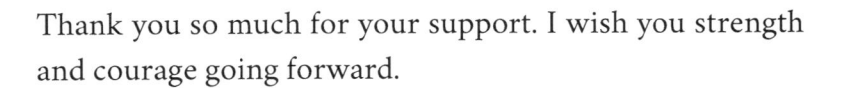

Thank you so much for your support. I wish you strength and courage going forward.

Scan the QR code below

REFERENCES

AARP. (2018, July 10). *Nutrition and dementia: How caregivers can improve mealtime*. AARP. https://www.aarp.org/caregiving/health/info-2018/dementia-nutrition-loss-of-appetite.html

Alzheimer's Association. (2022). *Home safety checklist*. https://www.alz.org/media/Documents/alzheimers-dementia-home-safety-checklist-ts.pdf

Alzheimer's Society. (2020). *Making your home dementia friendly*. https://www.alzheimers.org.uk/sites/default/files/migrate/downloads/making_your_home_dementia_friendly.pdf

Alzheimer's Association. (n.d.-a). *Communication and Alzheimer's*. Alzheimer's Disease and Dementia. https://www.alz.org/help-support/caregiving/daily-care/communications

Alzheimer's Association. (n.d.-b). *Daily care plan*. Alzheimer's Disease and Dementia. https://www.alz.org/help-support/caregiving/daily-care/daily-care-plan

Alzheimer's Association. (n.d.-c). *Dental care*. Alzheimer's Disease and Dementia. https://www.alz.org/help-support/caregiving/daily-care/dental-care

Alzheimer's Association. (n.d.-d). *Incontinence*. Alzheimer's Disease and Dementia. https://www.alz.org/help-support/caregiving/daily-care/incontinence

Alzheimer's Association. (n.d.-e). *Medication safety*. Alzheimer's Disease and Dementia. Retrieved September 5, 2023, from https://www.alz.org/help-support/caregiving/daily-care/medication-safety_(1)

Alzheimer's Association. (n.d.-f). *Tax deductions and credits*. Alzheimer's Disease and Dementia. Retrieved September 11, 2023, from https://www.alz.org/help-support/caregiving/financial-legal-planning/tax-deductions-credits

Alzheimer's Project. (2020, June 7). *The importance of routine and familiarity to persons with dementia*. Alzheimer's Project. https://alzheimer

sproject.org/the-importance-of-routine-and-familiarity-to-persons-with-dementia/

Alzheimer's Society. (n.d.-a). *Changes in eating habits and food preference.* Alzheimer's Society. https://www.alzheimers.org.uk/get-support/daily-living/changes-eating-habits-food-preference

Alzheimer's Society. (n.d.-b). *Communicating and dementia.* Alzheimer's Society. https://www.alzheimers.org.uk/about-dementia/symptoms-and-diagnosis/symptoms/communicating-and-dementia

Alzheimer's Society. (n.d.-c). *Daily care of teeth.* Alzheimer's Society. https://www.alzheimers.org.uk/get-support/daily-living/daily-care-teeth

Alzheimer's Society. (n.d.-d). *Dementia and language.* Alzheimer's Society. https://www.alzheimers.org.uk/about-dementia/symptoms-and-diagnosis/symptoms/dementia-and-language

Alzheimer's Society. (n.d.-e). *Dementia and sensory impairment: Communicating.* Alzheimer's Society. https://www.alzheimers.org.uk/about-dementia/symptoms-and-diagnosis/symptoms/communicating-dementia-sensory-impairment

Alzheimer's Society. (n.d.-f). *Drinking, hydration and dementia.* Alzheimer's Society. https://www.alzheimers.org.uk/get-support/daily-living/drinking-hydration

Alzheimer's Society. (n.d.-g). *Eating and drinking.* Alzheimer's Society. https://www.alzheimers.org.uk/get-support/daily-living/eating-drinking

Alzheimer's Society. (n.d.-h). *How physical and sensory difficulties can affect eating.* Alzheimer's Society. https://www.alzheimers.org.uk/get-support/daily-living/eating-physical-sensory-difficulties

Alzheimer's Society. (n.d.-i). *Improving the eating experience.* Alzheimer's Society. https://www.alzheimers.org.uk/get-support/daily-living/improving-eating-experience-dementia

Alzheimer's Society. (n.d.-j). *Poor appetite and dementia.* Alzheimer's Society. https://www.alzheimers.org.uk/get-support/daily-living/poor-appetite-dementia

Alzheimer's Society. (2019). *Recognising when someone is reaching the end of their life.* Alzheimer's Society. https://www.alzheimers.org.uk/get-support/help-dementia-care/recognising-when-someone-

REFERENCES | 157

reaching-end-their-life
Alzheimer's Society. (2021a, March 8). *How does dementia affect washing and dressing?* Alzheimer's Society. https://www.alzheimers.org.uk/get-support/daily-living/washing-dressing
Alzheimer's Society. (2021b, March 8). *How to support a person with dementia to get dressed or change clothes.* Alzheimer's Society. https://www.alzheimers.org.uk/get-support/daily-living/getting-dressed-changing-clothes
Alzheimer's Society. (2021c, March 8). *Personal grooming and dementia.* Alzheimer's Society. https://www.alzheimers.org.uk/get-support/daily-living/personal-grooming
Alzheimer's Society. (2021d, March 8). *When a person with dementia doesn't want to change their clothes or wash.* Alzheimer's Society. https://www.alzheimers.org.uk/get-support/daily-living/dementia-washing-changing-refusal
Alzheimer's Society. (2021e, September 2). *How to support a person with dementia to wash, bathe and shower.* Www.alzheimers.org.uk. https://www.alzheimers.org.uk/get-support/daily-living/washing-bathing-showering-tips
Alzheimer's Society. (2021f, September 3). *End of life care for a person with dementia.* Alzheimer's Society. https://www.alzheimers.org.uk/get-support/help-dementia-care/end-life-care-dementia
Alzheimer's Society. (2021g, December 20). *How to communicate with a person with dementia.* Alzheimer's Society. https://www.alzheimers.org.uk/about-dementia/symptoms-and-diagnosis/symptoms/how-to-communicate-dementia
Alzheimer's Society. (2022, January 19). *Non-verbal communication and dementia.* Alzheimer's Society. https://www.alzheimers.org.uk/about-dementia/symptoms-and-diagnosis/symptoms/non-verbal-communication-and-dementia
Alzheimer's Society. (2023, January 11). *What not to say to somebody with dementia.* Alzheimer's Society. https://www.alzheimers.org.uk/blog/language-dementia-what-not-to-say
Assal, F. (2019). History of dementia. *Frontiers of Neurology and Neuroscience, 44,* 118–126. https://doi.org/10.1159/000494959
Atkinson-Willes, B. (2021, November 29). *Reduce dementia agitation with*

a calm environment: 5 helpful tips. DailyCaring. https://dailycaring.com/reduce-dementia-agitation-with-a-calm-environment-5-helpful-tips/

Barbian, T. (2017, June). *The skill of patience.* Columbia Metropolitan Magazine. https://columbiametro.com/article/the-skill-of-patience/

Behrman, H. (2023, March 27). *Memory care help for families: Surprising ways to pay for care.* A Place For Mom. https://www.aplaceformom.com/caregiver-resources/articles/how-to-pay-memory-care

Better Health Channel. (2014, May 31). *Dementia - activities and exercise.* Better Health Channel. https://www.betterhealth.vic.gov.au/health/conditionsandtreatments/dementia-activities-and-exercise

Bloom, G. S. (2014). Amyloid-β and tau: The trigger and bullet in Alzheimer disease pathogenesis. *JAMA Neurology, 71*(4), 505–508. https://doi.org/10.1001/jamaneurol.2013.5847

Bryant, E. (2021, March 16). *Study reveals how APOE4 gene may increase risk for dementia.* National Institute on Aging. https://www.nia.nih.gov/news/study-reveals-how-apoe4-gene-may-increase-risk-dementia

Cherry, K. (2022, October 6). *10 ways to improve your resilience.* Verywell Mind. https://www.verywellmind.com/ways-to-become-more-resilient-2795063

Connolly, C. (2021, February 25). *10 ways to develop patience as a caregiver.* Guideposts. https://guideposts.org/positive-living/health-and-wellness/caregiving/family-caregiving/advice-for-caregivers/10-ways-to-develop-patience-as-a-caregiver/

DailyCaring Editorial Team. (2021, October 4). *Dementia communication techniques: Calm, positive body language.* DailyCaring. https://dailycaring.com/dementia-communication-techniques-calm-positive-body-language/

Eating & nutritional challenges in Alzheimer's disease. (2019, May 23). Cleveland Clinic. https://my.clevelandclinic.org/health/articles/9597-eating-and-nutritional-challenges-in-patients-with-alzheimers-disease-tips-for-caregivers

Family Caregiver Alliance. (2012). *Toileting (for dementia).* Family Caregiver Alliance. https://www.caregiver.org/resource/toileting-dementia/

Fowler, K. (2019, August 26). *The importance of self-care for caregivers.* A Place for Mom. https://www.aplaceformom.com/caregiver-resources/articles/the-importance-of-self-care-for-caregivers

Garcia, Lauren. "40 Inspirational Quotes for Caregivers." Care.com Resources. Last modified February 14, 2023. https://www.care.com/c/40-inspirational-caregiver-quotes/

Ghebrai, M. (2021, March 16). *23 best caregiver support groups online and in-person.* A Place For Mom. https://www.aplaceformom.com/caregiver-resources/articles/caregiver-support-groups

Gillette, H. (2023, March 3). *5 medications to avoid for people with dementia.* Healthline. https://www.healthline.com/health/dementia/dementia-medications-to-avoid

Hall, A. (2022, June 29). Caregiving is the ultimate relationship challenge. Here's how to reclaim your love and yourself through it all. *Forbes.* https://www.forbes.com/health/healthy-aging/caregiver-relationship-challenges/

HCA Dev. (2022, January 21). *Why is nonverbal communication crucial in dementia care?* Home Care Assistance Winnipeg, Manitoba. https://www.homecareassistancewinnipeg.ca/importance-of-non-verbal-communication-in-dementia-care/

Health in Aging Foundation. (2015). *Caregiver self-assessment questionnaire.* https://www.healthinaging.org/sites/default/files/media/pdf/Caregiver-Self-Assessment-Questionnaire.pdf

Hoopes, L. (2016, March 15). *Personal resilience: How to be resilient when you're a caregiver.* Crisis Prevention Institute; Crisis Prevention Institute. https://www.crisisprevention.com/Blog/personal-resilience

How to achieve work-life balance as a family caregiver. (2021, November 15). 24 Hour Home Care. https://www.24hrcares.com/resource-center/how-caregivers-can-achieve-work-life-balance

How to have patience with your patient. (2018, August 29). All Heart Home Care. https://www.allheartcare.com/how-to-have-patience-with-your-patient-7-tips-for-caregivers/

How to talk about end-of-life care when a loved one has Alzheimer's disease.

160 | REFERENCES

(2016, November 8). The Conversation Project. https://theconversationproject.org/tcp-blog/how-to-talk-about-end-of-life-care-when-a-loved-one-has-alzheimers-disease/

Kimrey, L. (2023, August 24). *Barriers to self-care & how to deal with them.* My Life Nurse. https://mylifenurse.com/thought-barriers-to-maintaining-self-care/

Kindness can transform someone's dark moment with a blaze of light. You'll never know how much your caring matters. Make a difference for another today. (n.d.). Random Acts of Kindness. https://www.randomactsofkindness.org/kindness-quotes/133-kindness-can-transform-someones-dark

Leo Buscaglia quotes. (n.d.). BrainyQuote. https://www.brainyquote.com/quotes/leo_buscaglia_106299

Lundberg, A. (2023a, June 7). *20 activities for dementia patients at home.* A Place For Mom. https://www.aplaceformom.com/caregiver-resources/articles/dementia-activities

Lundberg, A. (2023b, June 19). *List of drugs linked to dementia.* A Place for Mom. https://www.aplaceformom.com/caregiver-resources/articles/these-drugs-may-cause-memory-loss

Madison. (2022, August 10). *Home safety for dementia patients: Tips & resources.* Meetcaregivers.com. https://meetcaregivers.com/home-safety-for-dementia-patients/

Making a connection: Your guide to non verbal communication with dementia patients. (n.d.). Mariposa Training. Retrieved September 1, 2023, from https://www.mariposatraining.com/blog-posts/making-a-connection-your-guide-to-non-verbal-communication-with-dementia-patients

Marley, M. (2013, August 13). *5 things to never say to a person with Alzheimer's.* UsAgainstAlzheimer's. https://www.usagainstalzheimers.org/blog/5-things-never-say-person-alzheimers

MemoryLane Care Services. (n.d.). *Medication management and Alzheimer's.* MemoryLane Care Services. https://memorylanecareservices.org/medication-management-and-alzheimers/

Miller, K. (2016, December 6). *Communication requires patience, understanding.* Enidnews.com. https://www.enidnews.com/news/

local_news/communication-requires-patience-understanding/article_169c9d83-b559-554b-9c57-077bf307a565.html
National Institute on Aging. (2017a). *What are frontotemporal disorders?* National Institute on Aging. https://www.nia.nih.gov/health/what-are-frontotemporal-disorders
National Institute on Aging. (2017b, May 18). *Home safety checklist for Alzheimer's disease.* National Institute on Aging. https://www.nia.nih.gov/health/home-safety-checklist-alzheimers-disease
National Institute on Aging. (2021a). *Vascular dementia: Causes, symptoms, and treatments.* National Institute on Aging. https://www.nia.nih.gov/health/vascular-dementia
National Institute on Aging. (2021b). *What is dementia? Symptoms, types, and diagnosis.* National Institute on Aging. https://www.nia.nih.gov/health/what-is-dementia
National Institute on Aging. (2021c, July 29). *What is lewy body dementia? Causes, symptoms, and treatments.* National Institute on Aging. https://www.nia.nih.gov/health/what-lewy-body-dementia-causes-symptoms-and-treatments
National Institute on Aging. (2022, October 18). *What are the signs of Alzheimer's disease?* National Institute on Aging; National Institute on Aging. https://www.nia.nih.gov/health/what-are-signs-alzheimers-disease
Neundörfer, G. (2003). The discovery of Alzheimer's disease. *Dialogues in Clinical Neuroscience, 5*(1), 101. https://www.ncbi.nlm.nih.gov/pmc/articles/PMC3181715/
Patel, K. P., Wymer, D. T., Bhatia, V. K., Duara, R., & Rajadhyaksha, C. D. (2020). Multimodality imaging of dementia: Clinical importance and role of integrated anatomic and molecular imaging. *RadioGraphics, 40*(1), 200–222. https://doi.org/10.1148/rg.2020190070
Population Reference Bureau. (2023). *Fact sheet: U.S. dementia trends.* PRB. https://www.prb.org/resources/fact-sheet-u-s-dementia-trends/
A quote by Christopher K. Germer. (n.d.). Goodreads. Retrieved August 19, 2023, from https://www.goodreads.com/quotes/6870085-self-compassion-is-simply-giving-the-same-kindness-to-ourselves-that
A quote from golden son. (n.d.). Goodreads. Retrieved August 19, 2023,

from https://www.goodreads.com/quotes/5310441-home-isn-t-where-you-re-from-it-s-where-you-find-light

Ramirez, D. (2023, March 30). *Portable order for life-sustaining treatment (POLST)*. NerdWallet. https://www.nerdwallet.com/article/investing/estate-planning/polst-portable-order-life-sustaining-treatment

Reed-Guy, L. (2013, August 27). *The stages of dementia*. Healthline; Healthline Media. https://www.healthline.com/health/dementia/stages

Samuels, C. (2023, July 13). *Understanding the surprising costs of dementia care*. A Place For Mom. https://www.aplaceformom.com/caregiver-resources/articles/cost-of-dementia-care

SCIE. (2020). *Why nutrition is important in dementia*. Scie.org.uk. https://www.scie.org.uk/dementia/living-with-dementia/eating-well/importance-of-nutrition.asp

Singh, R., & Sadiq, N. M. (2023). *Cholinesterase inhibitors*. PubMed; StatPearls Publishing. https://www.ncbi.nlm.nih.gov/books/NBK544336

Stang, D. L. (2016, November 1). *"Hospice matters. The end of life deserves as much beauty, care and respect as the beginning."* SevenPonds Blog. https://blog.sevenponds.com/a-right-of-passage/hospice-matters-the-end-of-life-deserves-as-much-beauty-care-and-respect-as-the-beginning

The Light Program. (2017, June 13). *Importance of self care for caregivers*. The Light Program. https://thelightprogram.pyramidhealthcarepa.com/importance-self-care-caregivers/

35 inspirational quotes for caregivers. (2020, October 12). My Caring Plan. https://www.mycaringplan.com/blog/35-quotes-for-caregivers-thatll-brighten-your-day/

Tips for balancing life and caregiving. (2018, November 23). Best Care. https://bestcaremn.com/blog/balancing-life-caregiving/

Waterman, L. (2022, March 3). *The benefits of planning ahead for mums*. Women Who Win at Life. https://womenwhowinatlife.com/the-benefits-of-planning-ahead/

Waters, S. (2022, September 7). *6 self-care tips for caregivers*. BetterUp.com. https://www.betterup.com/blog/self-care-for-caregivers

Wei, M. (2018, October 17). *Self-care for the caregiver - harvard health blog.* Harvard Health Blog. https://www.health.harvard.edu/blog/self-care-for-the-caregiver-2018101715003

Why is self-care important for caregivers? (2019, September 5). 24hrcares.com. https://www.24hrcares.com/resource-center/self-care-caregiver

World Health Organization. (2023). *Dementia.* World Health Organization. https://www.who.int/news-room/fact-sheets/detail/dementia

Yang, H. D., Kim, D. H., Lee, S. B., & Young, L. D. (2016). History of Alzheimer's disease. *Dementia and Neurocognitive Disorders, 15*(4), 115. https://doi.org/10.12779/dnd.2016.15.4.115

Yu, D. (2021, June 7). *Eating and drinking difficulties in dementia.* BDA. https://www.bda.uk.com/resource/eating-and-drinking-difficulties-in-dementia.html

Printed in Great Britain
by Amazon